The Soul of

Caregiving

A Caregiver's Guide to Healing and Transformation

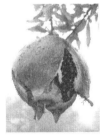

Revised Edition

Edward M. Smink, Ph.D.

The Soul of Caregiving: A Caregiver's Guide to Healing and Transformation – Revised Edition

Produced by Brian Schwartz for Wise Media Group
Cover Design by Tatiana Fernandez
Photo Credit: Nixson Borah

ATTENTION CORPORATIONS, UNIVERSITIES, COLLEGES, AND PROFESSIONAL ORGANIZATIONS:
Quantity discounts are available on bulk purchases of this book for educational or gift purposes. Special editions or book excerpts can also be created to fit specific needs.

Just as the pomegranate
reveals its inner secrets in
due season,
so too, does Soul refresh
with insight and wisdom.

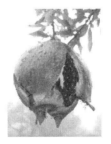

Why the Pomegranate?

The pomegranate is an ancient cultural symbol which has often represented fecundity and fertility. However, my love of the pomegranate comes from my spiritual roots with the Hospitaller Brothers of St. John of God, whose logo is a pomegranate. In the Judeo-Christian mythology, the pomegranate is a symbol of hospitality: the pomegranate opens itself, selflessly offering its seeds of eternal wisdom and hope.

Have you ever taken a bite of a pomegranate? Its bitter, crusty skin must be carefully peeled to discover the sweet, juicy, delicious seeds hidden within. Unfortunately, pieces of the skin are often stuck to the scrumptious seeds, leaving a bitter taste in your mouth.

I like to use the pomegranate as a metaphor for caregivers. In their daily work, they provide the sweetness of love, care, and compassion to those in need; however, like the pomegranate's bitter exterior, compassion fatigue can create a barrier that deprives the caregiver of their ability to acknowledge their feelings and tell their story, leaving them in a state of fear and isolation. But the painful bitterness of compassion fatigue can also alert the caregiver that it is time to seek help. This barrier must be removed gently, step by step, so that the caregiver's delectable seeds—their inner values, talents, attitudes, and strengths—can be refreshed, nourished, and celebrated.

As we slowly venture out of this global pandemic, it's important and necessary to reflect on our experiences. Since *The Soul of Caregiving* was published in 2018, many new insights have emerged, and the gradual accumulation of these new insights, ideas, and connections resulted in this revised edition. Throughout the reflection and revisioning process, I also learned more about the symbol of the pomegranate. Namely, I learned that the bitter taste of compassion fatigue can become an invitation to discover the sweet taste of compassion resilience, which leads to renewed energy, a greater life balance, and a rediscovery of the joy of caregiving.

Synopsis

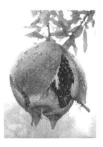

Who are the caregivers? We all are, for at the heart of being human is the capacity to care, to reach out to others and explore the relationships we build. *The Soul of Caregiving* is about us, and how we, as caregivers, serve, even sacrifice, for those in need. I invite you to explore with me how we can partake in a kind of sacred journey exploring our experiences as caregivers. Who will be your guide on this journey? Unlike other pilgrims who have a guide assigned to them, you will soon discover it is your own Soul guiding you. We may be professionally skilled to meet the needs of others, but we must also learn to stop and rest. It is not a waste of time, but rather, a necessity. We need time to ponder, reflect, and grow from our experiences. Not an easy endeavor amid a whirlwind of activity. We, as caregivers, experience vulnerability, helplessness, fears, and pain over the traumatic events we experience because we care. We care about those whom we are called to serve. Compassion fatigue arises because we care.

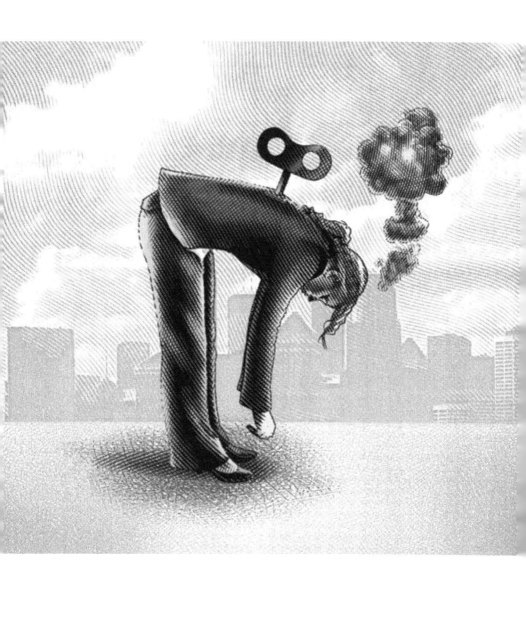

Praise for *The Soul of Caregiving*

The Consummate Guide for Self-Healing… A Must Read.

"Dr. Edward Smink brings new body and depth to his revision of *The Soul of Caregiving*. He compassionately and personally assures his readers there is a way to achieve the transformation needed to escape the darkness of compassion fatigue and burnout, and to re-enter into the light of well-being. Edward's clarity of expression, poignant and personal stories and reflective questions at the end of each chapter give his wisdom and insights credibility. This is a book of hope, vital to the resolution of a crisis, an important read for everyone."

William Devine, MA, Director of Graduate Admissions, John Jay College of Criminal Justice, CUNY (Retired)

"*The Soul of Caregiving* is a book for our time. Written as it is, by a nurse, a coach, and a spiritual director, Edward shares beautiful and touching stories from lived experience and compassionate insights for those suffering from compassion fatigue and burnout along with practical guidance for practicing self-care. The book is moving, pragmatic, and soulful, calling all of us who have responsibilities for others to recognize that care is a spiritual act as well as a courageous one. Ed wrote to me when I was experiencing compassion fatigue, reminding me of the cultural taboos against self-care. I was so touched by his kindness and helped by his insight that I posted it on my Facebook page and now I'm recommending his very fine book to you."

Carol S. Pearson, PhD, Author of *The Hero Within, Awakening the Heroes Within, and, most recently, What Stories Are You Living?*

"I had the great privilege and honor of crossing paths with Dr. Edward Smink when he blessed me with generosity, grace, and wisdom as a mentor on my journey writing about caregivers' burnout. *The Soul of Caregiving* is not just a book, it is a divine gift that has the potential to change and save lives of wounded healers across the globe. Edward puts his heart and soul into everything he does. His style of writing is elegant and deeply genuine. This book, I promise, will touch and transform your heart and soul."

Omar Reda, MD. Psychiatrist and Author of *The Wounded Healer*

"Dr. Smink's revised version of the ultimate guide for caregivers...*The Soul of Caregiving*...reinforced and strengthened my own personal commitment to take the time daily to step aside and continue to "peel the layers of the onion" by looking deep down inside of my own soul and with the shared insights, experiences, situations, advice and counsel of Dr. Smink... connect with my Higher Power. In doing so, I allowed for my own transformation and healing to move forward... and continue to evolve. This book was for me... a life vest that was offered to me at a time when I was drowning... and it saved my life. Let me say it once again... "*The Soul of Caregiving* helps you discover that God is not in what happens to you.... But God is found in what we DO with what happens to us" ... Being able to turn past hurts and disappointments into opportunities for redemption, is the "transformation" we have all been hungering for. I know it is true because it is happening to me."

Richard Hirbe, FSP, Masters of Pastoral Counseling, Board Certified Chaplain

"*The Soul of Caregiving* looks at caregiving in the broadest sense. Anyone who is in a caring role can relate to the stories and benefit from the reflections. I found it critical that I took the time to look at how I care for others and how that impacted me. Those of us who work with others on self-care need to remember to reflect on what we are doing for our self-care. I was so focused on care of others, family, and people I worked with, that I experienced severe Compassion Fatigue. I had difficulty believing what I was experiencing and was sure there was a medical reason for the way I felt. I finally reached out to my friend and coach, Edward, looking for his help. His book opened the door for me and I was ready to begin. Edward validated what I already knew, I had severe Compassion Fatigue. I had all the signs he discusses. I was forced to step back and focus on me and develop, once again, a plan for my self-care. It took me six months to feel I was in balance once again. I'd encourage anyone who is struggling to read Edward's book and seek a coach/guide to help you get back to health and wellness. "

Carol Schmekel, MHSA, BSN, RN, ACC, CENP, FACHE
Principal, Schmekel Coaching and Consulting

This book, *The Soul of Caregiving: A Caregiver's Guide to Healing and Transformation*, is the perfect companion for the road that we as caregivers are called to take--that of the person who accompanies a person who suffers. Accompaniment is a sacred calling, and one that requires us as caregivers to reflect on our own woundedness, our deeply held values, and our call to love those we serve. The Soul of Caregiving engages and challenges us to dare to move deeper into presence, both to ourselves and to others.

Christina Puchalski, MD, FACP, FAAHPM, Professor of
Medicine and Health Science, Director of The George
Washington University's Institute for Spirituality and Health
(GWISH), Author of *Time for Listening and Caring:*
Making Healthcare Whole

"As a 'caregiver' several times over (Nurse by training; primary caregiver for 89-year-old mom who recently died, suffering from dementia; spouse of someone with a life-threatening illness, leadership coach), it was easy for me to read Ed's stories and see myself within them. His prose, stories, quotes, and references to esteemed authors provides validation for our common humanity. Ed's integration of humor helped me to notice my own shadows, and embrace them with compassion, and light. Perhaps most importantly, Ed helped to bring into the light the common syndrome of "compassion fatigue" where we, as caregivers, may come face-to-face with our darkest shadow where we find anger, hostility, sarcasm, and aggression Ed normalizes these reactions and aptly reminds us to practice forgiveness. His courageous, personal illustrations where he showcases his own vulnerability remind us that we are in conversation with someone who's 'been there; done that.' *The Soul of Caregiving* is not a book to be rushed through. It is a non-judging companion that one could pick up during many phases of our life."

Joy W. Goldman RN, MS, PCC Certified Physician Development Coach Leadership/Executive Coach

"*The Soul of Caregiving* is a most meaningful work not only for those who are caregivers in the healthcare industry but for all those who willingly give themselves in many caregiving ways to make others feel better. The work is pleasantly and surprisingly engaging leading me and I hope other readers to pause and reflect on our special calling as a caregiver, of the sacred and transformative work that we do, and how we can build compassion resilience with self-care."

Dr. Tom Royer, MD. CEO and Partner, Royer-Maddox-Herron Advisors

"Caregiving requires an openness to one's own vulnerability, as one is with another. Facing, understanding, and embracing one's own brokenness is not a necessary hurdle to overcome for being an effective caregiver, but it is the very soul of heroic caregiving. Dr. Smink takes us on an incredibly rich and nuanced journey through the ages, evoking the sages of myths, symbols, psychology and spirituality to lead the reader along the redemptive mystery of caregiving and the inevitable call to self-truth and love at the heart of being not an effective but heroic caregiver. His "Timeout: A Moment of Reprieve - Time for a stop on the journey" at the end of each chapter provided ideal moments for honest self-appraisal and compassion. Thank you, Edward!

**David Lichter, D. Min. Executive Director,
National Association of Catholic Chaplains**

"I want to celebrate Dr. Smink's work. The first edition was an enormously useful and practical resource. The second edition proved to build on the utility of the first, which was grounded in fundamental truths, yet now provides a clarity and precision of understanding that helped me to appreciate the importance of taking better care of myself and the practical things I can do. After all, I am only human. In this edition, I held on to all that inspired me in the first edition, but now I know "the why" behind what I can do for me— so I can therefore effectively, and meaningfully, care for others. I learned, for example, that there are steps and actions I can take to heal myself so I can be more present and effective in my professional life, as well as in my personal life. Ultimately, at its core, this text celebrates the aspirations of human purpose."

**Dr. Christopher Cruz Cullari,
Professor of English and Education**

"In the *Soul of Caregiving*, Edward Smink shares his wise and compassionate voice with any and all caregivers (those born to the role, those who choose it as a profession, and those who come into it through life circumstances). He shares deep insights about the archetype of Caregiver--and helps any reader transform its trajectory in their lives from the potential for burnout and exhaustion to a more fully realized path of deep love for self and others. Stories and exercises throughout the book will help any caregiver relate to those on the same journey and reframe their experience as a redemptive and healing adventure. I highly recommend this book!"

Cindy Atlee, The Storybranding Group

"When I first read *The Soul of Caregiving*, I was drawn to the concept of "compassion fatigue" and the willingness to be open to the potential of a powerful and simultaneous reversal of roles, whereby the one in need, directly or indirectly, "heals [the] wounded caregiver." This passage aligns with my own experience since the 1970s. My husband of more than 50 years has suffered since his late 20s from an assortment of physically and progressively debilitating illnesses, primarily psoriatic arthritis. He's affected by all its devastating consequences, as well as an intolerance for most if not all medications available to alleviate the pain, immobilization and bone deterioration. And yet, he is unfailingly kind, selfless, filled with humor and a generosity of spirit, all of which indirectly inspires me every day to try to be a better person and act with deeper understanding and empathy in all ways. I also received this gift from him directly when I became seriously ill many years back and the role of caretaker was reversed. I have since fully recovered, but the lessons of his extraordinary empathy and kindness despite his own disability are with me forever. I'm grateful to Dr. Smink for affirming and bringing into focus the extraordinary power of empathy."

Pat Bennet, Author, Journalist, Home Caregiver

"I found this to be a unique book about caregiving. The author has spent his career in professional caregiving roles, and he draws upon this experience to deliver profound insights for other caregivers. The book carries a beautifully gentle and reassuring tone. I particularly enjoyed the discussion about caregiving as a spiritual practice. I believe that those who work in the helping professions--or anyone who is a caregiver at heart--will find this book to be especially rewarding."

**Dr. Aaron Bright, Professor, Author of *When Caregiving Calls*,
Founder of Caregiver Kinetics**

"As editor of the 2018 edition of *The Soul of Caregiving*, I found, as I was editing, that I was being transformed chapter by chapter. As a home caregiver for my father suffering from Alzheimer's, by the time he died, I was at my wit's end. My editing became a journey of recovery. Reflecting on the revised edition of *The Soul of Caregiving*, insights gleaned from my earlier editing continued to bring a more complete understanding of the step-by-step approach to recovery that I experienced from the trauma of caregiving. Edward's use of real-world stories to highlight the human aspects of the struggle and illustrate the many types of trauma caregivers face daily gives us, as it continues to give me, a path to reclaim our lives. This path enables the reader to move forward to recover from the negative, life-long effects of trauma and provides us with the inspiration needed to awaken our sleeping souls."

Rae McWhirter, Editor of *The Soul of Caregiving* (1st Edition)

Dedication

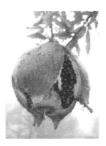

The journey of a caregiver is a heroic one, one that calls out of the caregiver a hospitality to serve, to be served, and to respond to those in need. It is a hospitality that gives voice to the unique stories of the host and the guest; it creates space to welcome and listen to the stirrings within one's Soul. I also dedicate this work to Mary, God's mother who has been a comfort and support throughout this journey.

To all caregivers, who tirelessly and selflessly give of themselves, and to all those with whom I have been privileged to serve, and who have taught me to be a caregiver, I dedicate this work. They have shaped and transformed me as a wounded healer, and they have helped me become a better and wiser person.

Dr. Edward M. Smink

Acknowledgements

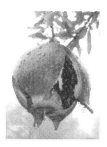

I am deeply grateful to my publishing consultant, Brian Schwartz, my previous editor, Rae McWhirter, and the editor of this Revised Edition, Daniel Siuba, who have guided me on this journey of publication and to Christine Downing PhD and Bill Devine MA, who assisted with editorial suggestions.

Secondly, I wish to thank the family and friends who encouraged and supported this endeavor, including Dr. Dennis Patrick Slattery, my literary mentor and guide.

I want to thank my partner, Dr. Nixson L. Borah, whose compassion, editorial voice, and support have guided me and made this book possible.

And finally, I am grateful for God's Spirit who has directed and guided me on the journey.

TABLE OF CONTENTS

The dance between the caregiver's needs and those of the one in need is explored. This chapter is an introduction to exploring something we do every day: to reflect on our experiences.

The question, "What is Soul?" is addressed, focusing on how the caregiver is empowered and sustained by going deeper into the inner caverns of one's being and listening to the inner beats of one's heart.

The magical and the universal underpinnings of the role of caregiving, in the broader mythic and archetypal realm of a culture, are examined.

Both the mythos and logos of caregiving is discussed. Each relates to faithless science and unscientific faith leading to a unity of the left and right brain functions.

This chapter explores how the caregiver, as host, experiences three different dimensions of hospitality: hosting the stranger, listening to the story of the guest, and understanding one's interior stirrings.

The ancient question of the frailty of humankind is explored. Within each of us is a space that seeks wholeness and transformation, an area of woundedness which seeks to be heard.

The art of reflection is a fundamental skill for caregivers which implies allowing the moment to take root and to reflect on how to nourish and sustain oneself as a caregiver.

Imagination helps one discover meaning and realize that the essential actions of a caregiver are spiritual.

What is a Practice? Is Caregiving a spiritual practice? These questions are explored as the ordinary becomes spiritual, as inner strengths and values give birth to meaning, insight, and transformation.

Compassion fatigue and its two sisters, secondary traumatic stress and burnout are examined. Caregivers experience compassion fatigue because they care.

Foreword

By Dennis Patrick Slattery, Ph.D.

Some years ago, Dr. Edward Smink invited me to write the "Foreword" to his new book, *The Soul of Caregiving: A Caregiver's Guide to Healing and Transformation*. I was, therefore, delighted to agree to Edward's request to write a second Foreword to a revised version of this popular text.

To be blunt: we need Edward's book, as well as his further expertise today, more than ever before. Not only individual souls are in crisis both in the United States and globally, but our national soul is suffering immensely from both the effects of repeated pandemics, and in the "mythic dissociation," a term from mythologist Joseph Campbell, suffered by many of our nation's leaders throughout our fragmented land.

Edward's term, "compassion fatigue," is a debilitating existential condition he has continued to explore in order to deepen his understanding in the intervening years. Moreover, as the author knows the power of stories in their intrinsic ability to connect us with one another, in this revision he has wisely expanded it to include more of his personal narrative. Such a move is a marvelous way to bring his material closer to home for all readers of this updated version.

I like and admire the fact that Edward was not content to simply patch together a new edition of *The Soul of Caregiving*. Rather, he continues to contemplate and broaden his world view on this therapeutic model. He has for instance, realized that caregivers "struggle with three cultural taboos that prevent them from developing skills of compassion and resilience: overcoming a lack of trust in one's self and others; lack of telling one's story and being heard; and the lack of dealing sufficiently with one's emotions."

As I muse over the values of this revision, I realize that Edward too has worked hard to further develop a sense of being "Present" to his clients and to those who serve others in their desire to become more whole and caring as individuals. He knows intuitively that an ego-centered approach to healing is bound to falter and fail. One must be present to the other in a far more wholistic way, one in which love for the other is the genesis for healing.

One's wounded soul life does not respond with much enthusiasm if the one addressing these lesions in the personality originates from a rigid model or an egoic position. Such wounding extends out to the caregiver him/herself. Being awake to the limits of one's own abilities is indeed a strength in relating to others who are in various degrees of crisis.

Caregivers are much more prone to be effective in actually helping another soul in crisis if they are freed from their own self-absorption in order to enter the dark woods of a person lost, dismembered or otherwise afflicted.

I have known Edward for many years and have observed his own deepening sense of who he is, with his enormous love that he shows for others; that in itself, when present to a client, is already a healing gesture towards their wholeness.

My hope for Edward is that this new vision of his capacities as healer and teacher will find a large audience. As he continues to teach and to work in this field that demands so much of him and others, the word of his excellent work, based on compassion and trust, the right individuals will continue to discover its treasures of insight. Those who come on his prescriptions for care will themselves be immensely rewarded.

Dennis Patrick Slattery, Ph.D.

Distinguished Professor Emeritus in Mythological Studies at Pacifica Graduate Institute and author, most recently, of *The Way of Myth: Stories' Subtle Wisdom.*

www.dennispatrickslattery.com

Introduction

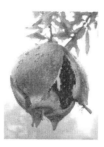

Revision is a common human practice. Said another way, revision asks us to adjust, to modify, and to change. Something each of us had to face as we explored seeing a new normal after over 18 months of adjusting to a worldwide pandemic. I experience some nostalgia over the past, and yet to be honest, I am becoming more conscious of the universal grief I experience with most of humankind. Three years ago, when *The Soul of Caregiving: A Caregiver's Guide to Healing and Transformation* was published, I was proud of the work and its reception. Life has its ways to season us to change and to adjust to a new normal that is nebulous and uncertain. I am tired of the pandemic and share with most a universal compassion fatigue. I know her symptoms well as one who suffered compassion fatigue twenty-five years ago. I had been painting the bars of my jail cell gold under the false assumption that the Soul Pain I was experiencing would just go away.

I, like any addict, found myself at rock bottom, like one lying in the gutter holding an empty whisky bottle, seeking to suck out the last drop. In the revised edition of this book, I have incorporated numerous insights gleaned over the past three years since its initial publication. These insights include a growing awareness of the cultural taboos that inhibit caregivers from seeking help, sharing their experiences, and allowing themselves to be vulnerable. I've also added new and updated research regarding compassion fatigue, burnout, and complex PTSD. And, perhaps most in keeping with the spirit of this book, I've integrated new insights derived from life experience, including reflections on both personal and professional experience. There are new stories illustrating the dynamism between the caregiver and the person receiving the care, as well as an overview in how other spiritual traditions embrace caregiving.

The vocation of caregiver is a deep and archetypal calling. It allows one to enter another's life in order to support them, often during periods of crisis. Caregivers witness and endure seemingly unbearable experiences. They stand firm and give life to those in need of care, even if their knees are shaking. In bearing what seems unbearable, the caregiver also experiences pain and suffering—they suffer precisely because they care. But who cares for the caregiver when they feel confused and overwhelmed? Who does the caregiver turn to when they feel alienated from their peers? Why do so many caregivers minimize their reactions to traumatic events and the vicarious suffering they experience? Why are caregivers afraid to reach out for help? These questions are central to *The Soul of Caregiving* and were part of the inspiration to write this book.

In my first edition, I reflected on a life of forty years as a caregiver in multiple healthcare and leadership roles. I felt as I do now, compelled to find my voice and let it be heard. There are many external reasons to write a book, but something deep within me ached to share the insights and wisdom which I hold as sacred treasures. I wanted to reach out to all who care selflessly for others. I wanted to assure them that the scars and interior wounds they've suffered as caregivers are invitations to rediscover their Soul. You are not alone, and you are not going mad when your soul aches because you have cared.

So, who are these caregivers? My definition of caregiving covers a diverse array of occupations and professions, including healthcare professionals, psychotherapists, certified coaches, chaplains, and spiritual leaders, as well as firefighters, police officers, and emergency medical personnel. I also consider active and retired military members, educators, parents, adult children who care for their parents, partners who care for each other, and political activists to be caregivers.

What is caregiving? It is a practice that requires focus, presence, and the ability to create a welcoming space for the one in need. In more extreme circumstances, the practice of caregiving requires the courage to act in dangerous, even life-threatening situations, but at its core, caregiving simply requires a caring heart.

This book is intended to create a space for readers to listen, become aware of, and claim their voice through the powerful act of reflection. This is not a "how to" book—it is an inspirational tool to encourage readers to turn toward their interior world. It is a book about rediscovering Soul, which is not a quick fix, but is more akin to a pilgrimage or journey which takes us beyond the surface, moves us deep into our pain, and gradually leads us to a reservoir of wisdom. This journey is both familiar and unfamiliar. It is laden with surprises and struggles, but ultimately results in insight, growth, and even healing.

It is my hope this book will inspire you to pause and reflect on your experiences of caregiving. I also hope it will help you expand and reframe the work of caregiving, situating it in archetypal, mythopoetic, and spiritual contexts. It is my wish that this book will both guide and support you as you continue to walk the path of caregiving. If you have the time, please write how the book affected you as a caregiver.

Many Thanks,

Dr. Edward M. Smink

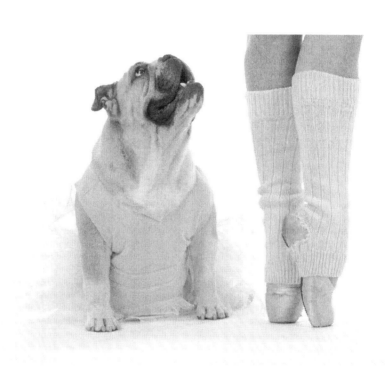

Chapter 1 - The Dance of Caregiving

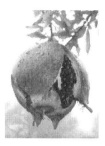

A Memory of Caregiving

We learn the art of caregiving from our life experiences. Sometimes, we learn this art before we even understand what we are doing. A childhood memory of mine illustrates this phenomenon.

I was six or seven years old, standing in my backyard. An abandoned puppy had wandered into our yard, and his bloody paw prints were etched in the snow. I knew he needed help, so I took him inside, extracted a piece of glass from his paw, cleaned off the blood, and bandaged the wound. I begged my parents to let me keep him, and they relented. I named him Sandy, and he became my first pet. This is my first memory of caregiving, and it serves as a precursor to my fifty years of experience as a nurse's aide, registered nurse, pastoral counselor, executive healthcare leader, and life coach. You may have had a similar childhood experience of caregiving, or perhaps you learned later in life, but either way, the act of caring—which I call the art of caregiving—transcends culture because caring is at the core of being human.

Although individuals working in caregiving careers are educated and trained for a unique role with corresponding skill set, there is an invisible archetypal pattern operating beneath the external manifestation of their specific caregiving role. This universal aspect of caregiving connects us as human beings, but also makes us susceptible to similar forms of suffering. One of the primary forms of caregiver suffering results from an unwillingness to be vulnerable and honest about painful caregiving experiences. I believe the tendency to avoid vulnerability is both implicitly and explicitly learned through social conditioning and cultural taboos.

Cultural Taboos

Marcia Carteret explained, "Individualistic cultures stress self-reliance, decision-making based on individual needs, and the right to a private life."[1] Ingrained within this paradigm is the belief that one is invincible and must rely only on one's individual abilities. In this sociocultural context, asking for help, expressing pain, and being emotionally vulnerable are considered taboo—they may be even perceived as forms of personal weakness. Many caregivers are fearful of trusting others and are unable to share their experiences and be attentive to their emotions and feelings as a result of these cultural taboos. This tension may be the same for caregivers living in collectivist or communal cultures. For example, a person living in an individualistic culture may resist the urge to ask for help because they think they should be entirely self-reliant, while a person from a collectivist or communal culture may resist the urge to express their individual suffering because they think it is a form of selfish or self-centered behavior. However, regardless of the differences between their beliefs, both individuals fear vulnerability, and the desire to express their pain clashes with cultural taboos and biases.

Most caregivers I know find it difficult to accept thanks for the work they do. They often say, "It was nothing," "I'm just doing my job," or "It's my responsibility as a parent, spouse, first responder, etc." Always vigilantly preparing for their next task, caregivers are notorious for emotionally distancing themselves from painful experiences—they tell themselves they are too busy to stop and listen to what is stirring within. Many say, "It's just too painful to go there." They also avoid sharing their experiences because they worry what their colleagues or friends will think. If they truthfully share how much an event impacted them, they fear others will think they are not capable of handling the work. They think they will be told they are not tough enough or strong enough to handle the job. If these fearful tendencies are reinforced, they gradually become unconscious patterns of behavior, like reflex responses. The caregiver's emotions and feelings become buried, which hinders their ability to debrief, feel, reflect, and ultimately heal from their painful experiences. These avoidant tendencies are first learned through sociocultural conditioning, but eventually the caregiver continues to perpetuate these avoidant patterns regardless of whether external forces pressure them to do so.

The caregiver's first step in formulating an antidote to these toxic beliefs and patterns of avoidance is allowing themselves enough space to slow down, pause, and consciously engage in the act of reflection.

Reflection

During significant life events, such as birthdays, anniversaries, graduations, marriages, divorces, deaths, and births, memories spontaneously flood our consciousness, as if asking to be revisited. Reflection is the process of turning inward and reviewing one's memories of an event, which can include reexperiencing emotions and feeling states, recalling or being unable to recall the chronological order of events, and potentially deriving new meanings or insights from the event. Sometimes, reflection can be like daydreaming—it can sweep us away to places of wonder and excitement. Other times, reflection is a gradual, slow process, like a seed germinating in fresh soil. As the seed dies to give birth to new life, we are often surprised by the insight and wisdom that result from its growth. Can you recall the feeling of being captivated by a child's laughter? Do you remember what it was like to experience the birth of your children and your grandchildren? At the birth of her first grandchildren, a set of twins, my sister remarked, "I thought I knew what love meant until I felt such love for these babies."

Life is full of vibrant and poignant moments which stir and awaken what is dormant within us. I still remember descending the spiral staircase of the Musée de l' Orangerie in Paris to view Monet's water lilies for the first time. I was not prepared for what happened next: as I entered the oval room and glimpsed Monet's water lilies, I felt myself enter a sacred space, like a cathedral. The water lilies, like stars in a darkening sky, broke through the canvas with a brilliance that captivated my Soul. In moments of reverie and reflection, time and space vanish; the present moment is transformed, and we witness a glimmer of the infinite.

Remembering beautiful moments can initiate the process of reflection, because it is easier to reflect upon experiences that were awe inspiring, pleasant, or were already meaningful to you. However, after becoming more comfortable with reflection, it is imperative that the caregiver begins to actively engage with memories and experiences that are decidedly unpleasant, confusing, or even chaotic. The unaddressed pain from these difficult experiences can be better understood as a deeper form of suffering called "Soul pain."[2]

Soul Pain

Michael Kearny, a physician in palliative care, explained Soul "points us inward and downward to the roots of our humanity and suggests that reconnection with our Soul is the central issue."[3] When we speak of the Soul, we speak of the psychic energy and life principle that sustains us. James Hillman, pioneer of archetypal psychology, described Soul as the "unknown component which makes meaning possible, [and] turns events into experiences."[4] Soul pain is like a signal that alerts us to listen to those interior voices that seek to be heard, acknowledged, and understood. Those voices may be speaking about painful events which yearn to be made into meaningful experiences. The presence of Soul pain also serves as an invitation to enter a journey toward healing. Pain sears our Soul when we witness unjust or unethical behavior, but Soul pain is also felt when we ignore our inner lives, which requires just as much care as our external lives. Soul pain reminds us that something within is screaming for our attention, and in order to address these voices, we must continually reconnect with ourselves and our Souls through the process of reflection.

The emotional strain of life and death situations experienced by paramedics and first responders may eventually take its toll in the psychological what is called complex posttraumatic stress disorder (PTSD), especially if disturbing or traumatizing events are not shared through group debriefing, counseling, or therapy. In less extreme circumstances, a caregiver may simply feel an uncomfortable emptiness stirring inside them. This stirring, common to all caregivers, is the sound of Soul pain echoing out, needing to be heard. Interior psychological walls built up for protection can be both supportive and isolating. These walls are like the skin of pomegranate—its tough, crusted skin is protective, but also hides the radiant, ruby seeds growing within; these seeds are our interior richness. Sometimes old walls need to crumble so that better, healthier boundaries can be established. Caregivers can learn to consciously create personal boundaries in collaboration with Soul, so that the entirety of their being is acknowledged and held in love and respect. A greater degree of psychological and emotional flexibility becomes possible, allowing the caregiver to gracefully move between their interior life and the exterior world. This oscillating movement between personal reflection and external action, via caregiving, is best imagined as a dance—the dance of caregiving.

The Dance of Caregiving

During my early years as a caregiver, I struggled with self-care. I did not know how to say "No," and because I was so busy helping others, I had little time for myself. Because I did not use my innate caregiving skills to nurture my emotional, psychological, and spiritual well-being, I succumbed to compassion fatigue and fell into the darkness of burnout. Sadly, this is not a unique experience for caregivers. The irony is that although caregivers are trained to listen, evaluate, and problem solve, they do not utilize these tools in their own lives and suffer as a result. What I call the Dance of Caregiving is a metaphor for the rhythmic movement between caring for others and caring for oneself.

The Dance of Caregiving is a dynamic balancing act which is maintained by our ongoing attention. This dance requires attunement and reflection, both during and after caregiving experiences. Risk-taking is involved, namely, the risk of vulnerability. Ironically, caregivers often take many risks for others but fear taking healthy risks on their own behalf. The caregiver must balance the tension between being present to the needs of the other while simultaneously remaining in contact with themselves.

Maintaining the continuity of this connection with yourself can help diminish the pain of the Soul. This process is not an "either/or" but rather a "both/and" experience. In this dance, our task is to learn how to listen and attend to both our own well-being and the wellness of others, before, during, and after caregiving experiences.

The Dance of Caregiving can lead one into the thrill of being absorbed in the music, the rhythm, and the interchange between partners. Dance consists of both individual and relational elements: on an individual level, each partner must know their steps, but on the relational level, each partner must be aware of the other, attentive to subtle movements, and emotionally receptive or assertive, depending on the needs of the moment. All of this requires the capacity to be present and aware of one's feet (perhaps you remember the awkward feeling of accidentally stepping on your partner's shoes). Caregivers, especially in crisis situations, need to focus on the unique situation at hand—there is little room for missed steps. However, too much focus on "what needs to be done," often leads to a rigidity, a lack of humor, and a resistance to reflection. Excessive focus can also result in forgetfulness—we can forget our dance partner, the music, and even the dance itself. In the Dance of Caregiving, maintaining an awareness of both inner and outer experience is crucial—too much emphasis on one or the other and we may step on our partner's feet, stumble, or even fall on our face.

A Story of Caregiving

People in crisis situations are often in shock; they have difficulty listening and making decisions. As caregivers in these situations, we are often forced to repeat ourselves, not because of a lack of interest by those affected, but because it is difficult to hear when one is in crisis. A nurse in the ICU once complained to me about a patient's family member who was having difficulty understanding her directions. Rather than judge the nurse or the family member, I used this moment as an opportunity for reflection—my colleague and I discussed the fact that our capacity to listen and process information becomes numbed during crisis situations. As caregivers, it is generally understood that our responsibility is to provide a safe, supportive space for the person in crisis, but we must also be patient.

We cannot force a person in crisis to understand our guidance or directives if they are incapable of hearing us.

A metaphor I often find helpful in explaining this process is the image of a parent instinctively embracing their tearful child. Reaching out with extended arms is another way of saying caregivers must create an external container of safety and reassurance for those we are called to serve. A personal story about a grieving couple in an emergency room provides a brief illustration of this kind of supportive containment, as well as an example of the Dance of Caregiving.

It was two days before Christmas. Jose, a young corpsman, and Angelica, his wife, were in a state of absolute shock. They had just lost their baby girl to sudden infant death syndrome (SIDS). They had planned to visit Angelica's family for Christmas, but instead of traveling as a family, they were being questioned by the police in order to rule out any wrongdoing in the sudden death of their infant daughter. Imagine the sensitivity needed to support this grieving family.

As I sat and listened to Jose and Angelica's story, my eyes filled with tears. The grief I felt could not be put into words, yet instead of being overwhelmed by it, I was able to contain the situation and help a grieving family understand the legal ramifications of SIDS. The combination of my formal training, as well as my experience healing from compassion fatigue and burnout, helped me to both understand and embody the Dance of Caregiving. I was able to support and contain Jose and Angelica without losing touch with my own emotional experience. I remained aware of my own feelings without letting them inhibit my ability to listen and be attentive to their needs. Without reflection, I would not have been able to maintain the balance between these two seemingly disparate worlds. Without the ability to reflect, listen, and respond to my own Soul pain, I could have easily become overwhelmed by Jose and Angelica's tragic situation. Or worse still, I would have continued to hold onto their grief and suffering for weeks, months, or even years after my involvement with them had ended.

The questions at the end of each chapter are meant to help you pause, still yourself, and reflect for a moment. You can engage with these questions however you like, but I would encourage you to take your time with each one and not rush the process.

A Moment of Reflection

1. Can you recall your earliest experience as a caregiver? How old were you? Who was involved? What happened?

2. Has revisiting this experience helped you understand something about yourself as a caregiver?

3. When you think of the word "reflection," what comes to mind?

4. Is taking time to reflect on you experience easy for you? Is it difficult?

5. Did any insights arise as you read this chapter?

_____

_____

_____

_____

_____

_____

_____

_____

_____

_____

_____

_____

_____

_____

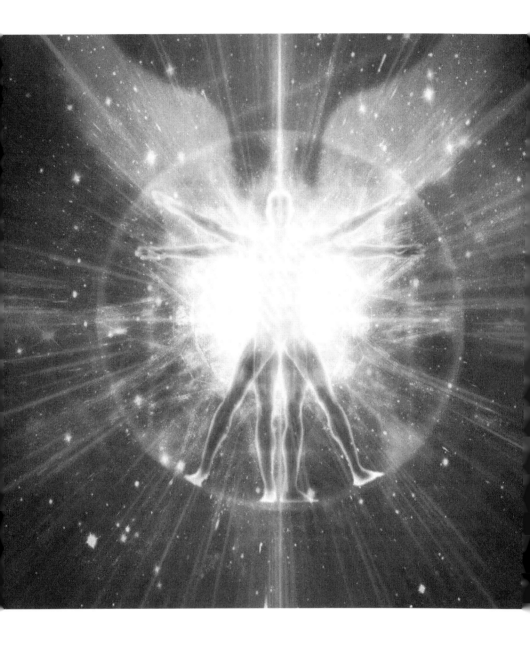

Chapter 2 - Reclaiming Soul

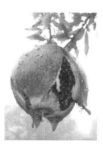

To understand the Soul of caregiving, we must first understand the nature of Soul. Simply put, Soul is an animating force—it enlivens us, our experience of the world, and each other. Even though we are taught to think of body and soul as separate entities, the living reality of a person is encompassed by both aspects of being.

Soul cannot be seen in its essence, but we can easily recognize its presence in our edible and audible creations: *soul food* and *soul music*. Soul is embedded in the way we describe solitary introspection and worldly exploration: we *soul search*. In particularly significant relationships, we say we have found the mate of our soul: our *soulmate*. There are soulful homes, soulful towns, and soulful cities. We say a person is soulful, that is, they are filled with Soul. Soulful people express themselves with ease through their body, speech, and actions. In the presence of the soulful, our sense of presence is heightened—the silence of these moment feels endless; time seems to stop.

Just as there is soulless work, there is *soulful work*. Contrary to the notion that a career is simply a way to make money, if Soul has a say in it, our work may be understood as a vocation—a call from Soul imploring us to engage with the world in a unique manner. Once Soul has called out to us, it will not be satisfied by anything other than what it has asked for. Whether Soul's call came from within or without, and whether it feels like a conscious or unconscious choice, caregivers often feel they have been summoned to fulfill their work from a force beyond themselves.

However, along the way, caregivers can lose sight of Soul. They begin to ignore the soulful voices within and the soulful symbols from without. If these caregivers do not reclaim the soulfulness of their existence, they may overlook the meaningful and potentially transformative encounters their day-to-day work offers them. If met with presence and receptivity, these soulful encounters can enliven and enrich their caregiving work and their overall well-being. Being open and responsive to Soul requires vulnerability and sensitivity, and if caregivers rigidly avoid reflecting on the past, anxiously fixate on the future, or both, they lose tremendous opportunities for Soul growth, because these opportunities only exist in the present moment.

Reclaiming Soul simply means becoming aware of and listening to the promptings of Soul that seek acknowledgement. These promptings may occur spontaneously and sporadically, yet at the same time, they linger. They need to be revisited, reflected upon, and sorted out; the insights derived from these promptings may inspire, challenge, cajole, and empower us. You may feel hesitant about following these stirrings and ask yourself, "Where is Soul trying to lead me?" But despite your reluctance, resistance, and fear, Soul will persist and inevitably lead you where you need to go, as long as you are—eventually—willing to follow. Never worry about being "too late in life" for a change—Soul's time is always the correct time for you.

At this juncture, interior and exterior promptings pose similar questions. Humbling yet empowering, you begin to experience yourself as you really are—not what your parents, spouse, friends, or culture demand or expect you to be. This knowledge, which is derived from the wholeness of your being, is something you can learn to trust. How do you know? Because you know.

Many years ago, I gave a presentation called "The Spirituality of Caregiving" at a regional meeting for nursing assistants and home-care aides. During the group discussion, one consistent theme emerged from the stories of the caregivers. Together we discovered the central animating force that motivated and sustained them in their work—it was all about Soul. They also acknowledged they had come to love the people they cared for. Initially, I approached this group as "the expert," but as I listened to their stories, I became a student. I came to give a simple presentation, but in return they gave me a life-altering experience. Spirituality and the spiritual dimension of caregiving are discussed more fully in Chapter 8.

The Multifaceted Soul

Thomas Moore said Soul connects one with depth, value, relatedness, heart, and personal substance.[5] Notice the multifaceted understanding of the functions of Soul, like the gem radiating different hues. In this section, I have elaborated on Moore's various facets of Soul, particularly regarding how their relationship to caregiving.

Depth: Soul connects us with depth, and when we go deep, our imagination becomes our guide, leading us into the land of mythos, creativity, and meaning making. Depth is associated with exploring the inner resources of our being which forge our values and beliefs. Hillman stated that when we go deep, "the Soul becomes involved. The logos of the Soul, psychology, implies the act of traveling the Soul's labyrinth in which we can never go deep enough."[6]

People who are not drawn to or interested in this kind of depth rarely enter caregiving professions, because caregiving professions are inherently deep. Whether you are an emergency medical technician trying to resuscitate someone who has overdosed or a social worker performing a wellness check on an abused child, being a professional caregiver is neither shallow nor superficial. Prepared or not, it plunges us into the deep well of human experience, which can quench our Soul's thirst—but it can also drown us if we are not careful. Staying in touch with the depth of caregiving provides sustenance to caregivers and nourishes Soul.

Values: Values can be personal, familial, cultural, religious, and historical. They are fundamental and often define who we are, both individually and collectively. They provide focus, direction, and accountability. Forged in the incubators of familial, cultural, and spiritual traditions, values are tested over time, handed down from one generation to the next, but do not become personal until they are consciously adopted. In terms of work, every profession has its own code of ethics with a commitment to uphold that code. Caregivers are committed to service, sometimes at their own risk, as is the case with first responders. We can also intuitively sense when caregivers do not value their work. For them, caregiving is simply a job. Perhaps they have somehow lost the spirit of their calling, or are ignoring another, truer calling. Their work is suffocated by routine and in some cases, indifference. Anthony's postoperative experience illustrates how both caregiver and client suffer when caregivers lose their connection to their calling and its respective values.

Anthony spent the night in the hospital and suffered from interrupted sleep due to a high temperature. By morning, his bed was drenched with sweat. A nurse stepped into Anthony's room, but only partially; she had one foot in the room, and one foot in the hallway. She hesitantly introduced herself, and Anthony told her about his bed being wet. "Oh, you are going home today, not to worry," she said. Then, Anthony asked if he could get out of bed to go to the bathroom. The nurse nodded yes, walked over and released the bed rail, then walked back to the opposite side of the room. Being a nurse himself, Anthony knew that after lying in bed for such a long time he would need assistance in getting up to prevent hypotension, dizziness and possibly fainting.

Anthony sat at the end of the bed, dangled his feet, and slowly stood up. As he walked to the bathroom, the nurse left, and a different nursing assistant arrived and asked how he was doing. This new nurse was much more engaging, unlike the nurse whose body language was distant and whose presence was unwelcoming. Anthony told her about his concerns regarding the damp bed especially because he knew he would not be discharged for several hours. Within seconds, the nurse remade his bed and Anthony's faith in caregiving was restored. Later, Anthony learned the first nurse was an agency nurse who was unfamiliar with the routine of the hospital. Her nursing mentor had also been sick that day. Regardless, the difference between these two caregivers is evident—one caregiver met Anthony with hesitancy and distance, and the other met him with hospitality and fearless engagement.

Relatedness: Relatedness, a desire to reach out beyond oneself, is at the heart of being human. We yearn to be in a relationship with the world, an intimate partner, friends, and family; we also yearn to be in relationship with ourselves and the transcendent Other. The philosopher Houston Smith described how the Islamic poet and mystic Rumi understood relatedness in a tripartite model. If we focus on the transcendent Other, we will inevitably discover something about ourselves and about creation. However, if we first reflect on the beauty of creation, which includes our friends and family, we may eventually experience the presence of the transcendent Other. Likewise, if we reflect on the miracle of who we are, we will discover something about creation and the transcendent Other. The very essence of Soul is to relate and to be in relationship.

Heart: Soul is about heart. Consider the Tin Man in *The Wizard of Oz*. He laments that he is "an empty kettle" who could be human "if he only had a heart." The hollow sound of an empty kettle epitomizes a lack of soulfulness, and therefore, a lack of humanity. Caregivers lacking in sensitivity, empathy, and compassion are disconnected from their heart. These individuals may be victims of the Age of Reason.

In the 17th century, English physician William Harvey performed one of the first autopsies during which he held a human heart in his hands. This surgical endeavor collectively transformed the heart from the metaphorical center of human love and compassion to a literal mechanical pump. When the heart became purely mechanical, the metaphorical and sacred dimension of the heart was lost. Hillman asked how all that the heart symbolizes, such as the courage to live, the center of one's strength and passion, love, feelings, the locus of one's Soul, and sense of person can be held in the hands of the physician or the coroner?

During the same historical period in which the heart became a pump, Hillman noted that a French Visitation nun, Margaret Mary Alocoque, had a mystical experience of Jesus as the Sacred Heart.[7]

In other words, the medical model that separated the heart from the sacred mystery of human love and compassion was balanced by the emerging vision of the archetypal heart, imaged as the Sacred Heart of Jesus. This is the heart that loves all of mankind and dissolves the illusion of a dualistic heart, body, spirit, and soul. In its deepest sense, the heart is at the center of every soulful encounter.

Personal Substance: Lastly, Soul is the very essence of being human. Substance implies a steadfastness of character and involves the most essential nature of our being. Robin, a nurse I greatly respected, shared a story which reaffirmed my sense that she was a deeply compassionate person with a strong character.

Robin was caring for a patient named John, whose doctor told her John's death was "Just a matter of time." John was the lone survivor of his family, and it was difficult for him to speak. John had already decided he did not want aggressive treatment and a "Do Not Resuscitate Order" (DNR) was already in place.

As Robin administered John's medications, she saw the sweat on his brow and the fear in his eyes. She wiped his face with a cool damp towel and freshened his pillow. Robin sat down next to John's bed and took his hand in hers. John smiled. Robin asked if he was comfortable, and he shrugged his shoulders. "Not so good?" she responded. Although no one had told him, Robin sensed John already knew the truth: he was dying. Robin, who had extensive experience working with dying patients, asked him, "Do you think God is calling you home?" John nodded and tears rolled down his face. Robin smiled, her own eyes a little misty. She gently nodded her head. There was no need for many words—they both knew what was happening. The fear melted from John's face, perhaps because he knew he was not alone. Robin and John both shared the belief that God was essentially compassionate and merciful, so in that moment, Robin asked John if he would like to pray together. He smiled and nodded his head.

As Robin began one of his favorite prayers, John followed along silently, only moving his lips as she spoke. When they finished, John was crying. Robin had other patients to check on, but promised John she would come back John after she finished her rounds. Robin assured John that a chaplain was already on his way to see him. Robin returned to John's room about 10 minutes later to find John lying peacefully in his bed. The chaplain told Robin that John had just died.

In reflecting on this story, I have often wondered about who was really guiding who. Certainly, John found Robin to be a guide and midwife in his journey of dying, yet almost thirty years later, Robin still talks about her experience with John.

The story of Robin and John encapsulates all aspects of soul, for it includes depth, value, relatedness, personal substance, and of course, a great deal of heart. Both Robin and John were present and open to each other, cried together, and prayed together. Robin gave John the gift of her loving attentiveness and support; John allowed Robin to share in and witness his peaceful, beautiful death. Certainly, both were changed by the experience at the deepest level, the level of Soul.

These multifaceted characteristics of the Soul radiate their specific hues "that point us inward and downward to the roots of our humanity and suggests that reconnection with depth is the central issue."[8] Soulfulness connotes an inner knowledge born out of the crucible of human experience.

A Collective Understanding of Soul

In addition to the individual experience of Soul, Soul can also be experienced in group encounters such as treatment teams, supervision groups, peer support, or debriefing sessions. The collective Soul of a group has its own needs and yearnings, which are subtly and overtly experienced by every group member. Like the phenomenon of Soul pain, the collective Soul of the group will cry out when something is out of balance and in need of attention. The team takes on a collective archetypal meaning which is more than the individual team. I witnessed some of the dynamics of the collective soul firsthand during a team building workshop I facilitated.

We began the workshop by reviewing the scores of the survey questions outlined in Patrick Lencioni's *Five Dysfunctions of a*

Team.[9] Lencioni's five dysfunctions are: Inattention to Results, Avoidance of Accountability, Lack of Commitment, Fear of Conflict, and Absence of Trust, and this team's scores demonstrated they needed improvement in all five domains. As I was reviewing them, one member expressed concerns about two or three members who were always late for team meetings. In response, I asked the group if they would like to address this issue. All agreed except for one member, who refused to commit to arriving on time, because she believed the needs of the patients should always take precedence. Although there was an obvious conflict of values, it was significant that the only person who could not commit to being on time was the same individual who was chronically late. Eventually, this team member confessed she deliberately came late because she did not value the team's collaborative efforts. It was a moment of serious Soul searching for the group.

As I engaged the group in a lively discussion, it became evident that although the group agreed teamwork was essential, they had not yet embodied this ideal or understood the importance of accountability and commitment. The group debated at length until finally I stood up entered the center of the circle. I drew an invisible line in the carpet with my foot and declared, "If you want to work as a team, you need to start right now. Otherwise, we are on a fool's errand." The group was stunned. Instead of continuing to debate their conflicting values, they became silent. I encouraged them to remain silent, to allow space for reflection and contemplation. Eventually, they agreed they needed to make a commitment to each other, for the sake of the team.

After the workshop concluded, I reflected on the moment I stepped into the circle to address the group's dysfunction. For me, that moment was completely spontaneous. Somehow, the collective Soul of the group took over and expressed itself through my words and my body. It implored the group to push through their resistance to commit to each other. By allowing the collective Soul to express itself, I was able to address the needs of the group in a very direct way. All I had to do was step out of the way and allow Soul to take over; then, the group members were able to come to an agreement.

Another significant moment of this workshop was the moment of silence that occurred after I entered the circle. The pause allowed for a moment of reverie, reflection, and stillness. These pauses are always available to us, but we usually do not stop and check in with ourselves until we are rattled by life circumstances or by the powerful words of another. True reflection requires commitment, consistency, and patience, and eventually produces self-confidence and empowerment.

A Time of Reverie

The lyrics of Simon and Garfunkel's song "Feeling Groovy" implore us to "slow down" because if "you move too fast" you cannot "make the moment last."[10] Making the moment last gives one permission to linger. In professional terms, lingering may take the form of what we call debriefing, which allows for individuals and groups to reflect on their experiences.

Lingering is Soul's way of acknowledging and listening to one's emotions, feelings, and inner knowledge. First responders know this all too well. They have nerves of steel yet contain hidden emotions which will later need attention (here lies the tension, the Dance of Caregiving described in Chapter One). Reverie allows time for lingering and dream-like meditation. It is a way of looking at what is real and then allowing oneself to entertain, free associate, and fantasize about these fanciful musings. As the sun illuminates the various facets of a crystal, so does this moment reveal all the different colors and hues that add to our stories and experiences.

Scholar of depth psychology Robert Romanyshyn suggested lingering allows one to experience the "invisible and subtle shapes and forms that shine through the visible, that sustain it and give it its holy terrors and its sensuous charms."[11] Many caregivers experience holy terrors coming into consciousness when they have time to linger, which is perhaps why they often avoid lingering altogether. However, lingering also creates the space to welcome that which Soul yearns to reveal. To linger is to embody a hospitable attitude which welcomes and accepts things as they are, without preconceptions or expectations. Hospitality is discussed in detail in Chapter Five.

Betwixt and Between

Soul has a certain perspective, a psychic viewpoint preceding all
other branches of knowledge. Soul is like a doorway, a threshold, an
opening between two spaces, but not a concrete place in and of itself.
For example, after we experience a psychologically disturbing or
emotionally overwhelming event, we are not immediately gifted
with insight and deep meaning. We may have been deeply affected
or even changed by what we experienced, but we must wait for
discernment. We must wait for answers to questions that are still
being formulated. This placeless place of waiting, this in-between
space, is the abode of Soul.

In an impatient culture that demands action and snap decision-
making, choosing to wait becomes a countercultural act. When we
learn to embrace the act of reflection and become familiar with the
patience and waiting that Soul searching requires, we learn to trust
our interior capacities, strengths, and insights. Gradually, we are
brought in touch with our inner resources and the underlying
patterns of our existence, which are called archetypes and archetypal
energies. Although the patterns themselves are invisible, they are
expressed and manifested in specific visible forms. In caregiving
professions, archetypes are made visible through unique forms of
service. To illustrate my point, I would like you to imagine two
scenarios.

First, imagine yourself speaking with a psychotherapist. You
meet with them in a quiet room, one on one, for fifty minutes. They
ask about your relationships, your childhood, and why you are
seeking therapy. During the session, they might say very little, but
they listen deeply to every word, gesture, and silence. Now, imagine
you are in a burning building, trapped inside a room. A firefighter
breaks down the door, and quickly ushers you out of the building,
away from danger. You will probably never learn each other's
names or see each other again. In these two scenarios, both the
psychotherapist and firefighter care deeply for you, but the form of
caring and the way it is expressed manifests in two entirely different
ways. Although they are both professional caregivers, two distinct
patterns of energy operate beneath the outward manifestation of
their external forms of service.

Archetypes are dynamic because they are not only rooted in ancient understandings of human experience but are also continually redefined throughout the ages. Contemporary nurses, firefighters, physicians, educators, chaplains, coaches, and safety officers might recognize that they carry on the traditions of generations past, but they must adapt these traditions to their current historical context. Archetypes are also alive in mythologies—not only in the collective understanding of a profession, but also in the individual myths each person brings to the profession. The archetypes of caregiving are discussed in detail Chapter Three.

A Moment of Reflection

1. How has your understanding of Soul changed after reading Chapter Two?

2. What insights have you discovered about yourself?

3. Has your understanding of being a caregiver changed? If so, describe it.

4. Have you ever experienced yourself in an "in-between" space? If so, what happened? How did it feel? What did you learn from the experience?

_____

_____

_____

_____

_____

_____

_____

_____

_____

_____

_____

_____

_____

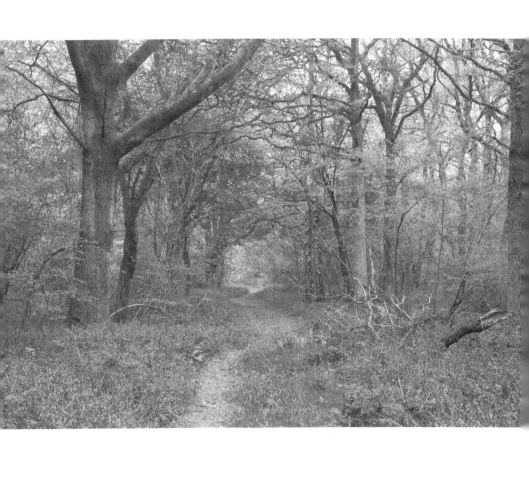

Chapter 3 - Caregiver Archetypes

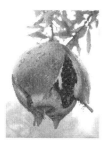

The Archetypal Imagination

In *Imagination is Reality,* poet and scholar Roberts Avens argued that imagination is the primal force and basic reality of human life.[12] Similarly, Jungian analysts Anne and Barry Ulanov suggested imagination "comes into play in all of our ways of being, in our thinking and feeling, in our intuiting, and our sensing. It expresses psychic life, which speaks first in images before it speaks in words."[13] The images that originate from deep within us, such as fantasies, dreams, and visions, are uniquely personal, yet they often follow universal patterns. These collective patterns are shared with past, present, and future generations of humanity. They are called archetypes.

Swiss psychiatrist C. G. Jung suggested an archetypal image is a primordial image which continually recurs throughout human history.[14] Consider the image of a flood. A flood is a naturally occurring weather event which can cleanse, destroy property, and claim lives. A flood can change the shape of an entire landscape. An individual might dream of a flood in response to an experience of being overwhelmed; the dream may also result from their psyche's need to cleanse or release something, and in the rarest of occurrences, may even predict an actual flood. But the flood also has collective, archetypal resonances. Images and stories about floods and flooding occur in collective historical repositories, such as religions, folktales, and mythologies. The contexts of these floods may differ, but beneath them lies the same invisible, archetypal structure.

Jung also described archetypes as those "factors and motifs that arrange the psychic elements into certain images, characterized as archetypal, but in such a way that they can be recognized only from the effects they produce."[15] Archetypes are both collective and individual as they reside beyond an individual as well as reside within the labyrinth of one's soul. In other words, we can recognize the effects of an archetype, but we cannot see the archetype directly. To stay with the core archetype of this book, consider the Caregiver. There are a multitude of examples of caregivers whose professions are influenced and shaped by social, cultural, and historical practices, but beneath their outward appearance and manifestation is the same invisible underlying pattern. This is the archetype of the Caregiver—the primordial pattern of caregiving, which is collective and universally shared. Even though its varying manifestations change throughout history, the same pattern continually manifests through us. For example, I have worked as a registered nurse, pastoral counselor, and executive healthcare leader, and though these are distinct professions with unique duties, I was able to utilize and express my caregiving capacities in each role. In other words, the clothing of the role may have changed from job to job, but beneath it, the body of the Caregiver remained constant, because each profession is an expression of Soul.

The patterns we often find ourselves embodying—or avoiding—have been outlined by scholars such as Carol S. Pearson, who identified twelve different archetypes.[16] These archetypes include the Caregiver, the Lover, the Hero, and the Explorer to name only a few. In this chapter, I examine the Caregiver archetype as well as its negative, shadowy form, the Caretaker. I also include a story about my experience of compassion fatigue and burnout, and the archetypal patterns that helped me heal from the experience.

Caregiver and Caretaker

Archetypes have many sides. They are like spectrums of rainbow light emanating a multitude of shades which are expressed and experienced by human beings as positive and negative qualities. The negative aspect or shadow side of the Caregiver is most evident in the form of the Caretaker. Caretaking is quite different from caregiving. The Caregiver is a deeply nourished by the soulful activity of caregiving; the Caretaker experiences caring as a repetitive and burdensome task which starves rather than feeds. The joy of caregiving becomes the task of caretaking. The Caregiver is relational and life-giving; the Caretaker is depersonalized and even resentful. Where the caregiver demonstrates compassion and concern motivating other to provide or be of service, the caretaker fails to connect people perspective with business outcomes. If the responsibilities of caregiving become a series of mind-numbing routines, something of the Soul is lost. Lost because the caregiver has been consumed by its shadow, the Caretaker.

When you become the Caretaker, life begins to feel very heavy. You sense that something is out of balance, and there is a loss of perspective. Adult children may feel this way when they begin to care for one or both parents. A sense of obligation obscures the joy of caregiving. Boundaries become blurred. In many families, the brunt of caregiving often becomes the responsibility of the female children rather than a shared responsibility of all the children. It becomes a breeding ground for resentment. Another shadow side of the caregiver may also be a perfectionist who needs to get everything done for others, and by doing so, neglects their own issues and needs.

Years ago, I read a book called *Addiction to Perfection* by Jungian analyst Marion Woodman. According to Woodman, perfectionistic behaviors result from the desire to meet unreachable goals and impossible ideals.[17] These behaviors, which are often obsessive and compulsive, are derived from a hunger for spiritual fulfillment. In perfectionism, spiritual hunger becomes psychologically displaced, and the perfectionistic individual repeatedly attempts to fulfill their spiritual hunger through overachieving, workaholism, and compulsive activity. I, along with many caregivers, lost my connection with my inner values and strengths. The Soul, the very core of our spirituality, is stifled and ignored, and the body, stressed and worked to exhaustion, pays a serious price.

In the next section, I tell the story of my descent into compassion fatigue and burnout, and my eventual return to the surface, which was achieved by utilizing the archetypes of the Explorer and the Hero to guide me back toward Soul.

The Slippery Slope of Compassion Fatigue

In every family, each member is assigned various roles which determine the overall structure and equilibrium of the family system. This applies whether the family is functional or dysfunctional—they both have a relative equilibrium. The roles are often assigned involuntarily and are usually based on the inherent qualities and capacities of each member in relation to the needs of the system, be it dysfunctional or healthy. According to Sharon Wegscheider-Cruse, an expert on addiction and codependency, each of these roles exacerbates the negative effects of the disease on each member of the alcoholic family.[18] Wegscheider-Cruse listed several roles played by each family member in the addicted family system, which included the addict, the enabler, the hero, the mascot, the lost child, and the scapegoat.[19] I mention these roles because I grew up in an alcoholic family system and became the Hero, the one who tries to bring the family together and create a sense of normalcy. Being the eldest child, I cleaned, gardened, and completed other chores behind the scenes. Unfortunately, the driving need to "do everything right" contributed to an extreme amount of pressure on me and left me susceptible to stress-related illnesses later in life. The groundwork for my slide into compassion fatigue as an adult had already been established early on in my life—I just wasn't conscious of it.

In Chapter One, I described my first caregiving experience when I told the story of meeting my dog Sandy for the first time, but within my family, I learned to embody the shadowy, negative side of the archetypal Caregiver: the Caretaker. A caregiver who feels invincible and does not develop skills of self-care gradually becomes a caretaker. Nourishing acts of caregiving become twisted into the burdensome, resentful tasks of caretaking which can harm both the caretaker and those they care for.

Caretaking became an unhealthy pattern which followed me into my adult life. I became extremely sensitive, even hypervigilant regarding the needs of others, and often neglected my own. Despite these unhealthy patterns, I still experienced moments of excitement and enthusiasm in my career as a registered nurse, pastoral counselor, and executive team leader, but neglecting my own needs came with a cost. Midway through my career, I experienced compassion fatigue, along with one of its sisters, burnout, which is called complex PTSD in clinical psychology research.

For three years, I was involved in a leadership development program for a non-profit charity. The winds of change were stirring, yet the organization was split down the middle, half wanting to go forward, and half resisting. Looking back, I did not take care of myself, nor did I realize I had organized my life in such a way that caring for myself became an impossible task. The inevitable whirlwind took me by surprise. I had little time for vacations or even days off, and I did not balance other responsibilities which I could have easily delayed or reassigned. The leaders of the program also nagged me whenever I requested time off. "Who has time for a vacation?" they asked. There was an attempt at conflict resolution, and I thought we were making some progress, but I still dismissed the internal conflict going on in me. I thought I was invincible, a common disease for caregivers. I forgot even Superman had an Achilles heel, kryptonite; a lack of self-care was mine. I lost my balance in the work and clouded over my natural instincts for caregiving. I had become a workaholic, but something was nagging at my gut, until one day, it all became too much.

Tears for Spaghetti Sauce

The dam eventually broke during a leadership conference I attended. Participants were asked to bring a potluck dish for lunch; it was sort of a community-building effort. As usual, I was late, and needed to put the final touches on the spaghetti dish I had partially prepared. I went to the kitchen to finish up cooking, and as I stirred the sauce, tears welled up in my eyes. Before I knew it, the tears became sobs, then a torrent. I broke down crying. The floodgates opened as I wailed, bent over in anguish. I knew I needed to add more water to the sauce—little did I expect it would come in the form of my tears.

I knew it then. I had had enough. There were too many conflicting events and situations, some bordering on abuse, some resulting from an utter lack of appreciation of my contributions, and my lack of understanding regarding my personal boundaries. My inability to say "No," and my need to take on more than I could handle finally brought me to tears. The well of caregiving had run dry. Shaking, I was barely able to tell the event coordinator I was not feeling well, and I left. I guess someone else served the spaghetti.

After this event, my recovery began. I started seeing a counselor, and I recognized I was suffering from compassion fatigue which was quickly sliding into burnout, which I now understand as complex PTSD. About one month into counseling, I asked my counselor, Leo, about the severity of my compassion fatigue: "On a scale from 1–10, with 10 being the worst, where am I right now?" Leo looked at me and compassionately said "Ed, you are between 8 and 9, and I consider 10 to be irreversible." I was stunned. Leo's response shocked me, but I was relieved I had sought help before it was too late. I had believed, yet again, that I was invincible until I learned I was not. The term "complex PTSD," manifested in me through my experience of Compassion Fatigue, took on a new meaning.

Previously, I thought PTSD was reserved for those who had experienced combat, but according to the National Center for PTSD, many traumas can lead to PTSD, including domestic violence, sexual or physical child abuse, terrorist attacks, physical or sexual assault, and natural disasters such as hurricanes, earthquakes, tornadoes, floods, and fires.[20] First responders witnessing traumatic events like a violent a car crash, a robbery, or violent attack are other examples of traumatic events. Both the individual experiencing the event and the individual witnessing the event can be potentially terrorized and subsequently traumatized.[21] In my case, I had experienced many traumatic events over many years, and though there were no physical guns, bullets, or bombs, there certainly were incidents of resentments, conflicts, unattainable expectations, violence, and emotional abuse.

After trudging through the darkness of compassion fatigue and burnout and finally attending counseling, I learned the importance of self-care. I removed myself from a painful living situation, changed careers, and gradually recovered. I would not have been able to make these changes if I had continued to embody only the strengths of the Caregiver. I had to call upon the strengths of other archetypal patterns in order to grow, heal and move forward. I had to let go of the negative side of the Caregiver, my caretaker role, as well as the shadow side of my hero, who was too pushy, failed to listen to other perspectives, and set the stakes too high. I also needed to rediscover and claim the archetype of the Explorer within me.

Reclaiming Soul

In order to heal from compassion fatigue and burnout, the central question is, "Can I shift from Caretaker to Caregiver? Is it possible to reclaim the inner spark within me, my soul?" Cindy Atlee of the Storybranding Group teaches an exercise to assist with this transition.[22] The exercise centers on creating balance for the Caregiver/Caretaker by allowing the strengths of the Hero archetype to emerge and relieve the inner tension created by too much reliance on the Caregiver archetype. In my career, I have observed that most caregivers have difficulty considering themselves to be heroes, yet when I ask if they think their work is, at times, heroic, they nod in agreement. Consider the courage of a firefighter rushing into a burning building, the risk a police officer takes in apprehending a criminal, or the parents of a chronically ill child who must continually cultivate a depth of compassion to care for their child every single day. The Hero or Warrior in each of us seeks to make a difference, to triumph over wrong, to meet an existing challenge. The strengths and values of the Hero are determination, courage, discipline, energy, principled action and giving your all.

So here is the dilemma. During our personal struggles, how do we recognize the shadow side of caregiving, and activate our hero's strengths? How many times do we need to be knocked off our horse to realize substantial action is necessary to recover from life as a codependent martyr? And if family dynamics led you into the role of an enabler, how do you use those same energies to care for yourself and establish personal, life-affirming boundaries? This is the mystery of it. Soul awakens you in transforming from survival to living. The energy you use to caretake and avoid is the same energy that can help you begin to truly live. Instead of the glass being half empty, the glass becomes half full. This shift in perspective allowed me to focus on all the caregiving experiences that nourished me in the past, as well as those that continue to nourish me today.

Years ago, during a class for my master's degree in counseling psychology, the professor told us that when we first start our personal journey, it often feels like being on a raft surrounded by sharks. He asked us to imagine a time we felt this way, then gave us a sheet of butcher paper and markers and asked us to draw the experience. I drew a broken whiskey bottle and reflected on being raised in an alcoholic family. As I mused on how I had survived, and how I had used so much energy to do so, I consciously became thankful for these energies. I said to myself, "Now, I want to use them to live." I no longer needed to be surrounded by sharks on a raft. Soul had awaken me and I found a way to go fishing instead.

Jung wrote that in every archetypal image "there is a little piece of human psychology and human fate, a remnant of the joys and sorrows that have been repeated countless times in our ancestral history."[23] Archetypes allow us, as caregivers, to experience belonging to a collective group larger than ourselves. There is a certain mythos that binds us to a group and whose membership gives us some standing in the agency and organization. But if we only call upon the qualities of a single archetype or, even worse, identify with the archetype itself, we lose the totality of who we are. If we identify solely with our caregiving qualities, we risk burning out and becoming fatigued, which can lead to the resentment of ourselves and of those we care for.

For me, it was necessary to learn I had other qualities beyond my caregiving capacities which could aid and support both my caregiving work and my life outside of my work. Recovering my Soul, the interior spark within me, guided me to make appropriate life choices. The person I am influences and unifies my professional and personal life. Learning to cultivate the heroic qualities of determination, discipline, and courage helped me to establish firm boundaries and to maintain those boundaries for the sake of my overall health and wellbeing. Another archetype, the Explorer or

Seeker, helped me envision new pathways, evaluate multiple options, define the most promising terrain, and make appropriate choices when necessary. I also had to struggle with leaving too many options open, and as the trail blazer, forgot to include others in what I was doing.

These archetypes, working in tandem with the Caregiver and influenced by Soul, helped me to regain a healthy level of control over my life. As I learned to take care of myself on every level—emotionally, physically, and spiritually—I began to enjoy my work and my life with a deeper fulfillment than I ever thought possible.

A Moment of Reflection

At your own pace, give yourself a moment of leisure to reflect on each question below.

1. On the spectrum from Caretaker to Caregiver, where do you find yourself?

2. How has your understanding of the archetype of the caregiver strengthened your resolve as a caregiver?

3. Can you give some examples of when you found yourself relying on these strengths?

4. What are your dreams about your profession? What gives you hope? What discourages you?

_____

_____

_____

_____

_____

_____

_____

_____

_____

_____

_____

_____

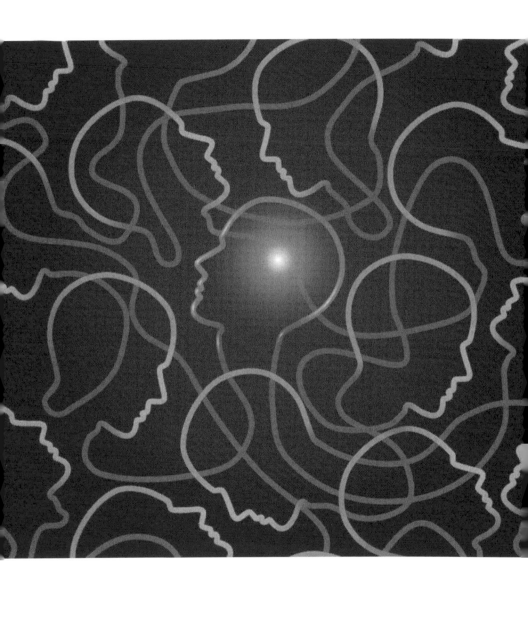

Chapter 4 - Truce and Consequences

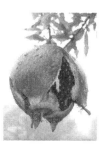

What if there were a truce between the right and the left hemispheres of the brain? What if these two very opposite functions really worked together? What would be the consequences if a balance or harmony existed between the mythos and logos, between the creative and the rational functions of the brain? Do they work separately or together? While the parts of the brain have different functions, they are designed to work together, as both halves play important roles in logical and intuitive thinking, in analytical and creative thinking.[24] Not either/or, but both/and, in this in-between space where one discovers their calling. I like this space, a space of reflection and insight, a place beyond the autopilot most caregivers experience. James Hillman asserted that within this space of questioning and discerning is the discovery of one's individual destiny, which is "between faithless science and unscientific faith."[25]

The Logos and Mythos of Science

Listen to these words of Hillman again, as they capture the essence of this chapter. "faithless science and unscientific faith." This was brought home to me when I was taking a class in anatomy and physiology in my nursing program at Newton Junior College. The red marks on my first lab report could have been etched in blood as far as I was concerned. The C- did not register well with me. I felt deflated. I thought I had done such a great job. Were these just delusions of grandeur? There seemed to be more red ink on the page than what I wrote. The uneasiness continued and found its way to the pit of my stomach. So, what was I going to do? Languish in self-pity, be the martyr, rally against the unfairness of the grade, or join a twelve-step program for students who felt they were victimized? Maybe that twelve-step program could be called "Misery-a-holics."

I cannot remember the exact moment when my left brain took over and simply asked the question, "What are you going to do about it?" Then, the right side of the brain suggested I be creative, as there were many possible solutions. Anything would be better than playing the victim. What did I need to learn? What was the scientific method all about, and how could I apply it to future lab reports? I remember looking at each part of the report that was underlined in red and made a note, as the blood was dry by now, maybe even coagulated. As I went through the report, I noticed the professor asked questions or add comments, which I recognized she didn't have to do. Rather, she took the time to do this because she cared. Each question and each note became the ladder for me to climb out of the hole I imagined myself in.

The Inquiry of Science

The scientific method is a framework of techniques utilized to carry out empirical research. A hypothesis is created, and the method of inquiry follows observation, measurement, and experimentation. This is the natural faith the scientist uses to analyze their hypothesis through testing and hopes for a predictable outcome. No transcendence here. The left-brain functions of analytic thought, logic, language, science, and math are alive and well.[26] Yet even in these moments that seem devoid of emotion, holistic thought, intuition, creativity, art, and music, are not these same scientists in awe when they trip upon something new, something unexpected, something laden with mystery that brings them to pause and reflect on what cannot be rationally explained? Welcome to the land of liminal space, the betwixt and between, a space of numinosity and mystery, which, if left unexplored, diminishes one's balance and perspective and leads to unfortunate consequences.

Tilly Was Her Name

Tilly was her name, a name that summed up who she was as a professor. I would describe her as colorful. Tilly was enthusiastic and passionate about teaching, with credentials in both science and the arts. Words were metaphors to her, and she would expound on how they brought life to science. Who would challenge us to move beyond the scientific fact, to the mystery related to it? The marriage of faithless science and unscientific faith.

In exploring the skeletal structure of the human body, Tilly's premise was, "Function dictates structure." She asked the class, "Why is there a bulge at the end of the femur, an area filled with spongy looking crevices, and how is this replicated in ancient and modern architecture?" The function of the bone is to carry weight, as are the various arches of a building. The more crevices, the more the weight can be distributed. Just look at the aqueducts of old, the ceilings of ancient times, the arches that distributed weight. The function—that is, to carry weight—dictated the structure. Even reminiscing about her, I chuckle over how much fun the class became. Every other report was an A or A+. Instead of being etched in red pen on paper or curdling blood as I imagined, the recommendations were carried by a company of neurons to be stored in my brain.

The Faithless Science of Logos: the logical, rational, verbal, linear, sequential, concrete forms of processing information. The Unscientific Faith of Mythos: the creative, intuitive, nonverbal, symbolic, seemingly random, holistic forms of processing information.[27] Overemphasizing one or the other leads to an imbalance or lack of perspective. In the following sections, I describe two examples which help to explore and illustrate this dilemma.

Julian's Task of Self-Care

Julian was a regional director of finance for a large healthcare system. When it came to numbers, balance sheets, and meeting deadlines, Julian was at the top of his game. Dressed impeccably with color coordinated socks, tie, and shirt, which contrasted his gray suit, he was tidier than his desk. He reminded me of a statistics professor (in my statistics class, only a notebook, textbook, and a pencil were allowed on our desks). Julian was crisp, clear, and clean.

As part of Julian's onboarding to the company, I was assigned to be his coach. When we began to discuss his goals, he told me the CEO asked him to explore his people skills. By "people skills," Julian meant the nonlinear, right-brain skills required to build relationships and cultivate positive social interactions. People skills were also related to his own self-care. The CEO believed that if Julian could understand how his own development of self-care would affect how he approached his staff and work, this would lead to a greater understanding of his peers and direct reports. Julian agreed he needed to explore how to develop his people skills. When he did take time to listen to what he was feeling, he recognized that lacking a sensitivity to his own needs caused a dull ache within him. He knew something was out of balance, and in a way, he was fortunate, for unlike so many others, he was aware of his own Soul pain. He wanted (well, sort of wanted or had a subtle inclination) to explore the relationship between developing goals around promoting his own self-care and how this affected his relationships at work.

As Julian and I were discussing his coaching goals, I introduced him to an article by Lisa McQuerrey called, "What are Good People Skills." McQuerrey's summary of these skills includes the ability to listen, communicate, and relate to others in a personal and professional way.[28] These skills extend to problem-solving abilities, empathy for others, and a willingness to work together towards the common good. We also explored some characteristics of self-care: it is not selfish, helps prevent burnout, builds relationships, and makes one more effective. Julian's homework was to review this article for our next session. Notice the interplay of the two horns of the dilemma for Julian: on the one hand, faithless science to get the job done, sacrificing all, including self-care, and his subsequent lack of focus on building relationships, which affected his people skills, and on the other hand, unscientific faith, the Soul pain that was gnawing from within to make a difference.

A metaphor for this dilemma is a person locked within a prison cell. The prisoner, who holds the key to the cell in their hands, chooses to stay locked inside. Instead of using the key, the prisoner paints the bars of his cell gold, believing that staying in prison is less painful than choosing to leave it. Of course, the opposite is true, as Julian spoke of his Soul pain while remaining locked in his workaholic prison.

In Julian's case, he needed to take one step at a time. He found it difficult to take time for self-care, as it conflicted with his current worldview. As much as he wanted to get started with coaching, he missed scheduled appointments, didn't do his homework, and gave excuses for not working toward his self-created goals. During one of our conversations, I guess the stars were in alignment. With all the red herrings filling the basket of my consciousness, and my desire to turn on the fan because of the smell, I resorted to tough love.

Several core competencies for my certification with the International Coaching Federation, of which I am certified as an associate coach, flashed before me: powerful questioning, direct communication, creating awareness, and designing actions.[29] "Julian," I asked, "what I am experiencing is a lot of excuses, or what I call red herrings. It is one thing for your company to assign a coach to all executive leaders, and for your boss to particularize his concern about developing your people skills, but coaching is most effective when you see the value of it for your personal and professional growth. In other words, do you really want to do this? Are you willing to explore with me the 'why' of your procrastination about taking steps to work on your goal of self-care? Are you willing to see how this relates to the understanding of your relationship to your own growth, as well as how it also relates to developing your people skills? It is all about relationships."

There was a long pause, and I knew there was a risk of Julian running down the hall telling his boss he did not need coaching. Julian caught his breath and said, "I'm very task-oriented and I like to get things done." Here was the faithless scientist, a mathematician to the core. Yet Julian continued speaking and shared he has a daily morning devotion which he does before coming to work. At first, I thought, "Another task on the list." Then he told me he reflects on the tasks that need to be accomplished for the day. He became animated as he shared how much this daily devotion, which he learned at his church, exhilarated him and gave him a perspective about his work. Julian then related the reason why he chose the company he was now working with: "I was impressed with their values and knew I could be at home here because of my own."

Now we are dealing with unscientific faith. I tried not to fall off my chair, as I was so pleasantly surprised and delighted. I got more than I bargained for from these direct and powerful questions. I had to put aside the temptation of fluttering my feathers like a peacock. It was not about me, but about Julian. I said, "Julian, I must admit, you pleasantly surprised me. I am delighted to hear how your devotion animates and directs the work you do. This is precisely the hope of your parent organization. May I make a suggestion? Why not make self-care one of your daily tasks? Your daily devotion is an indication that you do make time for self-care. Can you explore more ways?" A light bulb went on. He could add self-care to the list of his daily tasks. It worked. Julian learned to integrate his task-oriented skills with the creative and intuitive part of his brain. His coworkers and peers started to recognize a difference in how he related to them. He found the key to unlock the door of the prison he created, and now enjoyed developing this new skill.

Sarah & Maria: More Than a Late Report

Our next story begins with Sarah, who was the director of a large non-profit organization. One of Sarah's employees, Maria, a high achiever, failed to turn in a report that was due. Sarah was perplexed as this was very unusual for Maria, who had recently been hired. She had interviewed well and was highly recommended. Hiring highly skilled, professional women was one of the company's objectives, as well as Sarah's. In one of our weekly coaching sessions, Sarah asked how she should approach the situation. My immediate response was to ask what some of her options were.

Sarah's first response was to call Maria in and tell her how disappointed she was with her performance—linear thinking at its best. Yet, as she would realize later, there was a subconscious reason at play which added to her disappointment. Maria did not seem to fit Sarah's expectations of a professional woman. This was a learning experience for Sarah. She realized that in order to fully evaluate what was going on in Maria, she would have to put aside her expectations and disappointments. Then, Sarah told me she was personally concerned about Maria and wondered if there was something else going on. Sarah acknowledged her first approach was not going to work and wondered what she was going to do next. Together, we brainstormed in order to discover a more appropriate intervention.

Sarah genuinely cared for Maria (Yay for the right side of the brain!). I suggested she make an out-of-the-box executive decision to show her concern in a simple gesture. She decided to walk down the hall and visit Maria in her office. Sarah knocked on the office door and asked, "Maria, may I come in?" Maria said, "Yes, of course, please come in." Maria didn't expect Sarah to visit her. Sarah sat down, briefly discussed Maria's report, then asked: "Maria, how are you doing?" This question took Maria off guard, as she was expecting a reprimand. While appreciating the warmth of Sarah's concern, she was unable to allow it to sink in. Maria mentioned things were tough, but that she was ok, to which Sarah simply said, "I care about you, and I want you to succeed. Let me know if there is anything I can do," and returned to her office.

The next day, Maria knocked on Sarah's door and asked to speak with her. "Yes of course," Sarah responded and stood up to greet her. "Please sit down over there and I will join you." They sat next to a small table laden with fresh spring flowers, and Maria said, "Sarah, when you came by yesterday, I expected you to write me up and give me a reprimand. Instead, you warmly asked me how I was doing. I was caught off guard and needed more time to think it over. I needed to sleep on it. What I am going to tell you is difficult for me to admit and even harder for me to tell anyone else about. Sarah, I was recently diagnosed with breast cancer, and after a treatment last week, I had bouts of nausea, and felt sick most of the time. I was unable to concentrate fully on the report you asked me to complete." Maria's eyes filled with tears and Sarah reached out and held her hand. She knew her job was simply to listen, not to speak. Maria said, "I appreciated very much that you cared enough to see me yesterday. The fears I had about telling you about my diagnosis melted away. I am so grateful you took the initiative."

The treatment had made it difficult for Maria to concentrate on her job. It was even more difficult for her to tell Sarah about it until now. Sarah's intuition of caring was rewarded in trusting her concern for Maria. Unscientific faith is a person's ability to integrate business acumen with compassion. Sarah and Maria worked out a program and gave her additional collegial support, besides her own moral support. Maria recovered and is a trusted associate, as is Sarah, who learned the importance of showing a compassionate face and a new leadership skill. So, who coached who? They both did. Sarah and Maria coached each other.

Practical Applications for Caregivers

In a previous chapter, I asked, "Who are caregivers?" and answered, "We are all caregivers in one way or another." I have come to believe caregiving is at the heart of being human. Each of us has developed skills through hours of training—skills that are necessary to our particular profession or calling. These skills demand analytic thought, logic, use of language, and the logos of a situation. All of these are functions of the left side of the brain. I don't want a bicycle repairman taking out my appendix, nor do I want an untrained paramedic extracting me from an overturned car. When I arrive in the emergency room on a stretcher, my expectation is that I will receive competent and exceptional care from a group of highly trained healthcare professionals. Linear thinking, linear skills, and linear measurements help healthcare professionals make accurate diagnoses. Faithless science at its best. However, as important as linear thinking, training, and skills are, patient satisfaction scores consistently show that taking a moment to show concern and compassion are what most surveys rank as "exceptional care." A lack of these concerns ranks lower as "ordinary care" or even "bad care."

Angels to the Rescue

I am grateful for the emergency care I received after my car turned over on its side while on my way to a coaching session. Their skills were integrated with a real concern for me. I vividly remember telling myself to slow down and bear to the right as I traveled up a winding "S" curve road that cut through a hill. I remembered from other experiences cars barreling down the hill from the other direction. Then, all I remember is a kaleidoscopic canopy of trees and rocks entering my consciousness: multicolored images of weathered rocks and the massive black branches and green leaves of California silver oaks spinning. Apparently, as I was bearing to the right, my right fender hit the lower portion of the hill in such a way that the car flipped on its side. Perfect physics! As is true with most traumas, I blacked out. This experience is called traumatic amnesia.

Lying on my side with my seat belt intact, I was woken up by someone dressed in white (could it have been my guardian angel?) knocking on the window and telling me to turn off my motor. Like waking up from a stupor, sort of stunned, I said to myself, "Well this is a strange situation!" I reached for the button on the dashboard, turned off the motor, and then loosened my seat belt. Without my knowing it, a first responder climbed up and opened the passenger side door and asked if she could help me get out. I vaguely remember a hand reaching out to me as I stood up. I have no recollection getting out of the car. There I was, standing in the middle of the road, somewhat in a daze, gazing at the underbelly of the car; all the pipes, bolts, and wheel axles reminded me of the movie *Star Wars*. Suddenly, a woman appeared. She took out a white chair from the back of her truck and gently asked me to sit down. Later, I wondered, "How many people carry a white chair in the back of their trucks and appear at the right time?

A paramedic came over to examine me and encouraged me to go to the hospital to rule out a possible concussion. He was technically skilled, but he was also kind and concerned about how I was doing. Most of all, I remember his compassion. It was more than a job to him, and his people skills, his ability to listen and engage with me in a caring manner, were top notch. Sirens blaring, IV running, taking a blood smear to see if I was diabetic—I don't remember much else about the six-mile run to the hospital. Before I knew it, I was wheeled into an emergency room cubicle accompanied by the paramedics and an ER nurse. She was welcoming and reassuring, and as I would learn later, they were concerned I may have had a concussion. With some blood work, a trip to the x-ray department, and a thorough exam by the attending physician, I was good as new.

When I recounted the events of the accident to the hospital staff, they were all surprised I was not more seriously injured. In fact, when the results of the head x-rays returned, they were negative. I remember joking, "What did you expect? There was nothing up there anyway!" Again, I was impressed with their kindness and professionalism. Here was unscientific faith, where kindness, real compassion, and real people skills were practiced. While following their protocols, their care was exceptional. I was admitted for observation and released the next day.

In retrospect, I realize I was extremely fortunate. The accident could have been tragic. I could have been hit by an oncoming car, or my car could have started on fire, which would have been my demise. Though wearing a seatbelt was surely a factor in not getting seriously injured, I also believe it was those angels who saved me.

Too Busy to Care: Gloria's Story

One of the most frequent complaints of emergency room patients is that the healthcare professionals in the emergency room lack people skills. This is often the result of the triage system most emergency departments use to distinguish the most critical and life-threatening patients from those with less emergent needs. Often, emergency rooms become the public health agency of their city or county, as doctor's offices are closed, and urgent care centers are not available in a particular service area. Too much is asked of these dedicated professionals who must wrestle with priorities. Most of the time they get it right, as they did for me; however, the following story is about a time when they did not.

Gloria was working with her husband on a remodel of her kitchen. As they were tearing apart some cabinets, she slipped and stepped on one of the rusty nails sticking out from one of the torn studs. It was a Saturday afternoon, and Gloria became concerned about what to do. Remembering a friend who received a precautionary tetanus shot for a similar accident, she decided to search the internet for answers, and she discovered a tetanus shot had to be given within a certain time after the accident.

Realizing Monday would be too late to wait to see her doctor and knowing what the complications of not getting a shot could lead to, Gloria decided it was best to go to the ER to alleviate her fears. Unfortunately, it was a busy night. The triage nurse took the information, and since her situation was not emergent, she told Gloria she would have a long wait. The nurse was matter of fact and spoke in a monotone voice which communicated little empathy for what Gloria was feeling. "Non-emergent?" Gloria thought to herself, "But it *is* emergent. I don't want to risk the complications of not getting the shot." They each had a different view of what emergent meant.

On the one hand, the nurse was correct. Gloria was not having a stroke, bleeding to death, or having a heart attack, so in her view, this could have been handled at an urgent care center. True, but it was Saturday night and the urgent care centers were closed. On the other hand, the nurse could have acknowledged the seriousness of the situation, calmed Gloria's fears, and reassured her that she would do her best to make the wait as short as possible. For Gloria, this was an emergent situation, otherwise she would not have come to the ER. The task of the triage nurse was to evaluate the seriousness of the situation and decide when Gloria could see the doctor—job done, logic, and left brain to be awarded. But with a little more empathy, the situation could have been handled better, as discussed above. Instead of feeling calmed or reassured, Gloria began to fume because of how the nurse treated her. "Crusty and proficient to the core," she thought.

Later, when a survey about her experience in the ER arrived in the mail, she gave them a low score.[30] Needless to say, the hospital's administration was not pleased, as their ER scores were declining. In response to these scores, the hospital put an action plan into place and a fast track was developed within the ER.

Suck it up, Baby, Twist, and Shout

My experience as a healthcare professional has taught me most caregivers face a particular dilemma. They go from call to call, case

73

Edward M. Smink, Ph.D.

to case, meeting one need after another. They tend to "stuff" their feelings down or "suck it up" because they must move on to the next call, the next incident, the next whatever, especially in emergent situations. Caregivers build walls to protect themselves, and yet these same walls often separate and can distance them from those they are called to serve. These walls also prevent the caregiver from listening to those interior movements seeking attention, as well as doing the necessary debriefing on what is being felt. These responses hearken back to the cultural taboos mentioned in Chapter One: caregivers are fearful of asking for help, believe they are invincible, and think they must be completely self-reliant. This leads to a lack of trusting themselves, their teammates, and their families. This lack of trust hinders their ability to reach out and share their story with another. It's not advice they want—I know from my own experience that caregivers simply want to be heard. They have a story to tell. Not trusting and not talking about our experiences separates us even more for those we love as we bottle up our emotions and feelings. Onerous beliefs such as "boys don't cry" and "girls are too emotional" are seared into our unconscious minds. We stuff down and repress our emotions until we feel numb, but in doing so, we become more like a ticking time bomb ready to go off at any time.

Normal Feelings

Caregivers often forget they are going to experience emotions and feelings in response to whatever is going on around them and that these feelings are legitimate and even important. Contrary to the perception among caregivers that they must protect themselves from their emotions, caregivers are human beings with the same emotions and feelings as everyone else. I have come to believe this is the reason they shut down. What is being felt during a traumatic event is a normal reaction to an abnormal situation. There is an interplay at work between faithless science and unscientific faith, between the Logos of protection, the left-brain function, and the Mythos of creativity, the right brain function. Protection, which is related to survival, prioritizes logical, rational, linear, sequential, and concrete processing. The creative, compassionate, non-verbal, symbolic, random, and holistic processing, which intuits and imagines alternative possibilities, often takes a secondary role. The miracle is that these functions are integrated actions of both the left and right hemispheres of the brain, but all too often, caregivers overemphasize the logical, left-brained survival functions and lose touch with the creative potential and compassionate function of their right-brain, potentially resulting in an imbalanced perspective, compassion fatigue, and burnout.

I Felt Alone

Allison is a member of EMS (Emergency Medical Service) who was called to the crash of a twin-engine plane where the pilot was trapped. The pilot had radioed that he was having engine trouble before the crash. By the time she and her team arrived, the plane was engulfed in flames. Flashing red and yellow lights against the background of billowing plumes of gray cindered smoke, the smell of gasoline, and orange flames spewing towards the sky greeted the EMS team. Firefighters sprayed foam that resembled a washing machine overflowing and going awry. But it was too late, too hot, too dangerous to make an attempt to save the pilot. The cockpit was already filled with flames.

Every fiber of her body tightened as Allison witnessed what seemed to be impossible. Fight or flight responses at a standstill, caught in the liminal space of non-action. Skills, training, hours of preparation, could not have changed the situation. Their training taught them not to put their own lives at risk when any action they could have taken would be futile. "I just stood there, fixated and almost frozen" Allison recalls, "standing there in horror and staring at him in the flames. He was still in a seated position like he was driving a car. I stared and stared, it was all I could do. And all of a sudden, he took his last breath, his body slowly fell forward and rested on the controls," Allison, with tears in her eyes said that all they could do was watch the pilot hunch over and die. They could do nothing. Frozen in the moment of horror and hopelessness. "We are trained to do all that is possible to save lives and here for a moment that seemed like hours, we stood paralyzed in our inability to do anything."

Because they cared, each member of the team felt hopeless, stunned, and numb. What if they arrived earlier? What if the plane didn't explode? What if the pilot was less injured upon impact and could get out? Again, normal reactions to an abnormal traumatic event. Allison still recalls the face of a firefighter walking around like a zombie. He was pale and sweaty, and no one could talk to him. He was just gone. No one could do anything. Feelings, she admitted, were stirring within her. Feelings Allison would later admit were fear, guilt, grief, and hopelessness. Allison didn't recognize at first, the impact this event would have on her. Her emotions had shut down. Traumatic amnesia is a wonderful gift, as Allison did not remember much about the incident for a week or so. Then she told me that she was moody, even bitchy, and didn't sleep well. She snapped at the smallest things and didn't understand why. She would cry at the drop of a hat and screamed at her fiancé when he suggested that he wanted to take flying lessons.

A First Responder's Dilemma

The commander set up a voluntary debriefing for the team according to the ICISF protocols.[42] Reluctantly, Allison decided to attend, fighting the decision up to the day of the meeting, "Why the hell do I need this?" While not remembering all the details of the debriefing, she recalled that all the members of her team were experiencing the same reactions that she was. "I wasn't crazy, and I felt not so alone." Allison felt such a sigh of relief. Her team members were moody, drinking heavily, and not sleeping, experiencing emotions just as she was.

As first responders, Allison, like her teammates, when asked "How are you doing?" would answer "Fine, Just Fine," a first responder's code with a double meaning: The first means keep your distance because I am not going to get involved with debriefing and join what was commonly known as the "Cry Babies Club." A real conundrum, being strong at all costs, able to handle the situation by one's self, stuck in the cultural milieu of "I can handle this," and the real experience of being vulnerable. Allison mentioned that first responders often use the anagram F.I.N.E to disguise what they are really feeling. F.I.N.E. means "FUCKED UP, INSECURE, NEEDY, and EMOTIONAL."

Allison knew she really needed help. Having stuffed her feelings, and for whatever reasons, now she was ready to seek help. She knew that the other alternative would be a slow burn to self-destruction. This traumatic event shook her and the team to the core of their being. It left them all speechless and in shock because they experienced normal reactions to an abnormal, traumatic, and horrific event. I simply cannot imagine how I would cope with a similar situation. The symptoms of PTSD were setting in, which often occur within 72 hours after experiencing a traumatic event. It would take Alison years to recognize she was suffering from post-traumatic stress and then do something about it.

Conclusion

One of the requirements for my MA in counseling psychology was to have a personal therapist during the two-year program, as well as a supervisor in my practice hours of counseling. Research had shown, that while one is learning theory, at the same time, during the practice of counseling, personal issues would and could emerge where one needed a resource for debriefing and self-reflection. It was not an option. This was a degree requirement. Not an either/or, but a both/and where the activities of the left and right hemispheres of the brain worked together.[42] As discussed, there are a lot of "what ifs" after a traumatic event. What if these "what ifs" were a way that could be turned around to develop a new paradigm shift within the organization.

What if caregivers had a similar requirement during their training? That is, the recognition that they were going to experience normal reactions to abnormal traumatic situations. Instead of considering debriefing in what some would call "The Crybabies Club," or that one is not strong enough. What if debriefing was the normal routine instead of being hit and miss? Surely the outcome would be a stronger support team that not only had each other's back, but also normalized the human need for reflection and support. Would this not also increase employee satisfaction, decrease turnover, and sick days? I am reminded of an example I used in employee orientation. I had great fun using a commercial from the California Milk Advisory Board that always gives me a chuckle. The focus is that happy employees increase client satisfaction, as well as reduce complaints, and empower the customers that they serve. While it is about cows and cheese, the metaphor is obvious. "Great cheese comes from happy cows. Happy Cows come from California. Real California Cheese."[43] Happy caregivers and happy clients!

What if caregivers were given the opportunity that "the new normal" would be a more effective way of developing emotional intelligence, instead of the bias that debriefing is secret, abnormal, or a club for crybabies? Would there be more empowerment and better relationships with each other and their supervisors? Would there be less of a willingness just to "hold on" until retirement, and most importantly, less fear that one could develop compassion fatigue, burnout, or compound PTSD. Finally, studies have shown that happy employees increase client satisfaction, reduce turnover, and lower costs.[44]

Caregivers often experience the angst of wishing to improve their skills and wanting to be better both personally and professionally. Often one feels stuck, so to say, overwhelmed with too many choices that leads one to confusion and non-action. Often the fear of change or the unknown of what one would experience or feel appears to be more painful and fearful than opening the door. Caregivers often dull their interior pain, and paint, as I like to call it, the bars of their cells gold. As did Allison. The person she was becoming frightened her more than taking the risk to open the door of the jail cell that the traumatic event created. Understanding this process of being present to both inner and outer resources is the subject of our next chapter, Chapter Five: *The Ins and Outs of Hospitality* in which we focus on the interior attitude of hospitality.

A Moment of Reflection

At your own pace, give yourself a moment of leisure to reflect on each question below.

1. Although we are a combination of the different functions of the brain, what is your most prominent function, and how does it affect your work as a caregiver?

2. Of all the stories in this chapter, which do you identify with the most?

3. What practical goals could you set to improve self-care for yourself? Can you imagine some suggestions that would help improve the self-care skills of your colleagues?

4. What do you find difficult about debriefing after traumatic situations?

_____

_____

_____

_____

_____

_____

_____

_____

_____

_____

_____

Hospitality

an ancient word
which means both
host and guest.

Its meaning holds the
promise of sharing
the best of what we have.

It is a word overflowing
with abundance
like the pomegranate —
a rich ruby fruit from the desert
to comfort and
to delight.

Sister M Madeleina cy

Chapter 5 - The Ins and Outs of Hospitality

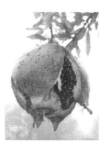

The ins and outs of hospitality involves an exploration of creating both inner and outer space, conscious and unconscious musings like breathing in and breathing out. Interior musings alert one to practice the acts of hospitality, an ancient word which means both host and guest reaching outward to the stranger. Ancient cultures understood the importance of being host to the stranger, as in many cases it meant the very survival of the guest. This was the norm in many societies, and the responsibilities for both host and guest were clearly outlined and commonly understood. Protected by the host, the guest was treated with respect, fed, sheltered, and considered a temporary part of the tribe or clan. The host and guest were equals.

Hospitality is Universal

In ancient Greece, hospitality was a right, and the host was expected to make sure the needs of the guest were met. A person's ability to abide by the laws of hospitality determined nobility and social standing.[31] The Sanskrit adage, "Atithi Devo Bhava," which means "the guest is truly your god," dictates the respect granted to guests in India. From a Hindu perspective, the practice of graciousness towards a guest comes from the belief that the guest was either favored by the gods or was a god themselves, and in offering hospitality, the host would find favor.[32] The Hebrew Scriptures tell stories of hospitality, such as when Abraham hosted three visitors

(Genesis 18:1ff), and when Lot and his wife offered hospitality to two strangers (Genesis 19:1ff). Noteworthy is how universal, if not archetypal, the theme of hospitality is in the history of humankind. The guests of Abraham and Lot are angels, representing the sacred, divine God. At the beginning of the Common Era, the Roman poet Ovid retells a Greek myth about Baucus and Philemon who are hosts to two gods, Jupiter and Mercury, who are disguised as humans.[33]

The stories in Genesis and in Ovid's *Metamorphoses* tell us Lot and his Wife, as well as Baucus and Philemon, were favored because they offered hospitality, unlike the parsimonious citizens who rejected their need for shelter and safety. Each story describes how the guests were welcomed and offered the customs of hospitality, such as the ritual custom of foot washing, being fed with a meal specifically reserved for honored guests, and of course, being given shelter. Because of their generosity and graciousness, Baucus and Philemon and Lot and his wife were blessed and saved from the destruction of their towns, whose residents refused to grant hospitality to the strangers.

In early Christianity, it was a common belief that in welcoming a stranger, you may be welcoming a god. By practicing hospitality in welcoming the stranger, you would be blessed. This practice is both praised and enumerated among the works of charity by which humankind will be judged. Matthew speaks about the rewards of the just, related to the Son of Man: "I was a stranger and you welcomed me" (Mat.25:35ff). Jesus had no home and was frequently a guest, as is mentioned throughout the Christian Scriptures.[34] Recall the story of Jesus rebuking Simon, his host, because he did not offer Jesus the customary rituals of hospitality, even in preparation for his death. These rituals were the obligation of Simon: to wash Jesus' feet and offer him the customary welcome for a guest.[35] When Paul and Barnabas were ministering to the citizens of Lystra, the crowds shouted "The gods have come down to us in human form,"[36] and later in Jerusalem, Paul exhorted the Hebrew community: "Do not neglect to show hospitality to strangers, for by doing that, some have entertained angels without knowing it."[37]

Archetypal Underpinnings of Hospitality

I want to explore the ancient belief that when the host offers hospitality to a stranger, he may be entertaining an angel or a god. This insight is central to our discussion, because I believe our work as caregivers is both transformational and sacred. In our numerous acts of hospitality, of creating inner space to welcome the stranger, we, as caregivers, are given opportunities to ignite the sacred spark of life within us. We meet the sacred in the other and in doing so, discover the sacred in ourselves. Pastoral counselor William Augsburger discussed this interplay between the caregiver and the one being cared for, which I believe is another fundamental attitude for the host. When the host is sensitive to the needs or wounds of the stranger, there is an interplay, a building of trust, and the experience of compassion. Likewise, as the host becomes an agent of healing, "when healing calls to healing," there is awareness, insight, repentance, change, as well as growth, and the host is transformed.[38]

This interplay has a way of moving us out of ourselves and into our common humanity. Understanding the practicalities of being a host is paramount to being a caregiver. Caregivers are hypervigilant in their readiness to offer hospitality to those in need. Caregivers practice hospitality par excellence each time they create the space to welcome a stranger. So universal is this act of hospitality that during national emergencies such as floods, hurricanes, and fires, first responders and volunteers act without hesitation, responding to the stranger in danger. Even those affected reach out to their neighbors to offer support and safety. As host, being hospitable is about being welcoming, open, and receptive—actions that are focused on another, as in welcoming a guest or a stranger.

Whether a stranger appears in the emergency room, at the scene of a crime, or in a burning building, caregivers, by their act of caregiving, train to be hospitable. In the words of Sister Madelina, "Hospitality holds the promise of sharing the best of what we have."[39] Giving the best also demands a discipline that, at times, is challenged and strained. How often have you heard the phrase "the client [or patient] comes first," or "the client [or patient] is always right," even if they are wrong? This attitude raises a multitude of conflicting feelings. How does a caregiver cope with these difficult and painful situations? How often do these situations challenge our core beliefs?

The story of Charles, a chaplain at a large medical center, provides another example of how to sort out challenging feelings in a tragic situation. Chaplains, too, need time to debrief, and in this story, we learn that it is possible to share and express the difficult emotions stirred up by a challenging caregiving experience through an act of creativity.

Grandpa, I Can't Play Football

Guillermo, a two-year-old boy, lay in a coma on a ventilator in the intensive care unit (ICU). The doctor called a family conference to discuss the child's dire prognosis and plan of care. Gathered in the ICU conference room were chaplain Charles Guillermo's doctor, and Guillermo's parents, Anita and Billy. The child's grandfather, Sergio, was also present. Sergio spoke of all the dreams he had for Guillermo and how proud he was to be his grandfather.

Guillermo was adventurous as any two-year-old. He was interested in the outdoors and loved to be in the family pool with his parents. On this summer day, his mother was busy with some friends and relatives planning Guillermo's second birthday party. One of the cousins was charged to keep an eye on Guillermo. Somehow, Guillermo wandered into the kitchen and saw the surface of the pool glimmering through the locked screen door. He wanted to go swimming and, determined as any two-year-old can be, jumped up and unhinged the lock on the door.

Meanwhile, the party guests laughed and giggled in the living room. For several minutes, no one seemed to notice Guillermo's absence. Then, someone cried, "Where is Guillermo?" They searched the house to no avail. They even looked under the bed where Guillermo often hid, but he was nowhere to be found. Then, they noticed the latch on the kitchen door was unhinged; terrified, they searched the yard and discovered Guillermo lying on the bottom of the pool. The paramedics could not find a heartbeat but still tried to revive him. He had a faint brainwave and was medivacked to the hospital by helicopter.

Since Guillermo was found without a heartbeat, and because he was underwater for at least thirty minutes, it was doubtful he would survive. However, Guillermo did survive, as children often do, but he sustained severe brain damage. The family agreed to continue treatment and hoped for the best. Each member of the support team personally felt the tragedy of this family, especially those who had children of their own.

The next day, the chaplain held a debriefing at the patient-care rounds with the staff. When it was his turn to share, Charles explained he was able to sort out his feelings by writing in his journal. Writing about the emotions he felt often helped him debrief, especially in situations that were too difficult to bear. As he journaled, a poem emerged, which he shared with the group. It was called "Grandpa, I can't play football anymore." Here is his poem.

"Grandpa, I can't play football anymore"

Each time Guillermo's eye caught the reflection of glimmering light, he ran for the pool. Young, energetic, he was always stopped by a guardian who knew the danger of a two-year-old toddler falling into a swimming pool.

Doors locked, watchful eyes, careful to harness the energy of Guillermo who forgot he could not live in water.

Careful each moment, except one moment that changed everything. All the dreams, all the hopes, all the wishes of a family changed that afternoon when Guillermo thought he was a fish.

A visitor to the door, a mix-up in who was watching a curious thunderbolt, and thunderbolt he did, out the door and into the pool. Thirty minutes he laid there, on the bottom. Life being pushed out of him by the displacement of air for water.

"Where's Guillermo?" The scream of a mother and family members. 911 and drugs and CPR as dedicated first responders cannot change that moment.

His grandfather sighs, his dreams lost for his only male grandson who lives only minimally, whose loss of oxygen leaves him in a deep coma.

In the silence, in the unspoken words and unfocused look, he thinks he hears a voice:

"Grandpa, I can't play football anymore."

The Different Faces of Hospitality

Creating space for the other allows the host to entertain a curiosity about the client's story, a willingness to be receptive to their fears, anxieties, and concerns. This second dimension of hospitality deals with the caregiver's skill and practice of active listening in further understanding the stranger's needs.

I remember listening attentively while one of my professors addressed the importance of active listening during one of my courses in pastoral counseling. She said there are three rules that are the foundation of a great coach, caregiver, or counselor. "The first rule," she said, "is to listen." "The second rule," she said, "is to listen." Then she paused, allowing silence to activate the class' curiosity. She regained a quizzical poise, appearing whimsical and a little mischievous as she gazed at each member of the class. Finally, she broke the silence and said, "Can you guess what the third rule is in developing the skill of active listening? It is to listen!"

Although there are a variety of definitions for active listening, I like the one posted for diplomats on the U.S. Department of State website, which provides a visual metaphor, in the form of a Chinese character, that symbolizes the act of listening. The Chinese character tells us that to listen we must use both ears, watch and maintain eye contact, give undivided attention, and be empathetic. The article further states there are four rules to active listening, which explain the deeper meaning of the Chinese symbol: 1) to seek to understand before you seek to be understood, 2) to be non-judgmental, 3) to give the individual your undivided attention, and 4) to use silence effectively.[40]

In discussions of hospitality, much has been said about creating space for others, but little attention has been given to the inner promptings that the act of hospitality stirs within the caregiver. Promptings and feelings can both increase and deplete a caregiver's energies. The third understanding of hospitality focuses on the interior stirrings of the caregiver. Simply put, what do caregivers experience and how do they address these promptings and feelings? These can range from feelings of endearment, excitement, satisfaction, and joy over a job well done, to feelings of vigilance, caution, suspicion, hopelessness, anxiety, fear, and compassion fatigue. Hospitality is about tending to another, and at the same time, listening to the interior promptings of one's own Soul.

In summary, the three dimensions of hospitality are responding to a need, understanding what the client is experiencing, and understanding how you as a caregiver are affected. Inner and outer space seem to merge whether one begins with the need of another or with oneself.

Lost in Reverie

My earliest understanding of the ins and outs hospitality surprised me. It was the summer I turned thirteen. In hindsight, I found myself being host to the stranger within me who I had often neglected. I was too young and inexperienced to fully understand these interior promptings of my Soul. At the time, they were strange to me.

I was with my father and brother. We were on an errand to get our car serviced. My father's friend owned an auto repair shop in front of a set of railroad tracks. Car talk did not interest me, and after we toured the car shop, we learned it would take at least an hour for the car to be serviced. At some point, I must have wandered off on my own, creeping past the garage and walking up a hill that overlooked the railroad tracks.

I sat in a grassy spot on the hill, feeling contented. The abandoned railroad track meandered through the edge of town. Varying shades of gravel created a bed that cushioned the creosote-covered railroad ties, ties that fastened and held the rusted colored tracks. I wondered when the last train had passed through. I tried to imagine where it was going and where it came from. Then, I imagined myself sitting on a trestle with my feet dangling in the air. In that moment, I entered a threshold between what was before and what would happen next, an in-between place.

What drew me there, I do not know. I can only speculate. Maybe it was my love of trains (at home, I had two 4' x 8' sheets of green painted plywood in the attic, adorned with trestles, roads, houses, and a tunnel through a papier-mâché mountain). Maybe it was the wanderlust of travel, moving beyond a geographical boundary springing from the depths of my ancestral and immigrant past? Maybe it was simply an opportunity just to be, a moment of reverie, a common teenage escape.

I was focused on outer space, the warmth of the summer day, the freshness of the grass, wildflowers covering the hill, and the blossoming of new foliage on the nearby grounds. My attention was also on the tracks leading to nowhere—or was it somewhere I wished I could go? As I focused on the railroad tracks, I had become lost in a moment of wonder and reverie, drawn into my interior world, as if led by a mantra. It was as if I had been transported to an inner world of wonder and peace. Time vanished, and for a moment, I felt like I touched infinity. Even as I write, the experience continues to deepen within me, a feeling of transcendence and oneness.

For the first time in my life, I experienced Soul. Time ceased to exist. I was simply present in the here and now. In this juxtaposition of outer space and inner space, the two became one. I was too young, however, to glean any wisdom from this experience or to understand the stirrings of my Soul. It would take years for me to fathom the depths of this new awareness. After all, I had my turbulent teenage years before me, during which I struggled to understand my place in the world. Those years, tumultuous as they were, gradually led me to discover my calling as a caregiver.

Inner and Outer Worlds

I was very much in touch with my surroundings on that spring day. I cannot say I was in touch with my inner world, nor did I know how to relate it to the rest of my life. In exploring inner and outer worlds, where does one begin? Caregivers are drawn to respond to those in need, trained as it were, to be self-sufficient, almost on autopilot, walking a tightrope between these two worlds. The worlds of a doctor, nurse, caregiver, firefighter, police officer, paramedic, parent, and educator transcend any one participant. Their struggle is humankind's struggle to develop a relationship to interior and exterior resources, which reveals something about the mystery of being human.

Inner and outer worlds create inner and outer space, an openness to receive the story and experience of the stranger, an openness to the universe, and an openness to the movements of one's Soul. According to Sister Madelina, "Hospitality is a word overflowing with abundance, like the pomegranate, a rich and ruby fruit from the desert, to comfort and delight."[41] Pomegranates, like some caregivers, are crusty and hard on the outside; then, when the time is right, they open, becoming vulnerable and revealing their inner secrets. The pomegranate is an ancient symbol of fertility and charity, a metaphor for self-giving, of giving oneself completely. As the pomegranate reveals its inner secrets in due season, so too, does Soul refresh with wisdom and insight, a tagline I use in this book. When we become aware and listen, Soul refreshes us with wisdom and insight.

This is the paradox of exploring inner and outer space. The outer leads to the inner and the inner leads to the outer. The task for the caregiver is learning that the core of hospitality begins with oneself in the "in between space" where inner and outer worlds meet, which I call the betwixt and between of liminal space. Paraphrasing the words of Psalm 139 from the Hebrew Bible, if we go to the highest heavens or descend to the netherworld, take the wings of the morning or dwell in the deepest regions of the sea, or think we can hide in the shadows of the night, still the sacred spark of life, the unity of who we are, where inner and outer space meet, will be with us and in us.[42]

The mythologist Joseph Campbell expanded this notion of integrating inner and outer worlds in a discussion he had with one of his students. Campbell was exploring the ancient myths and religious traditions of monotheism and polytheism when one of his students asked, "Where does God live?" Campbell, somewhat amused, responded, "Is it above? Then the birds will be there before you. Is it below? Then the fish will be there before you. The Kingdom of God is within you. Who and what is in Heaven? God is in Heaven. Where is God? Within you!"[43] Think for a moment—what did you learn from your parents and religious teachers? Did they teach you God is in the heavens, in creation, in one another, in your imagination, or in your heart?

Campbell, as best he could, provided an example for his students (and his readers) to reflect on the mystery of the divine. It is an ancient question that continues to permeate the hearts of humankind where the sacred is experienced both within and without ourselves.

Experience as Teacher

My experience and awareness of hospitality became real when I joined a community of brothers who took a vow of hospitality. For over five hundred years, the Hospitaller Brothers of St. John of God developed monastery hospitals, clinics, and health centers for the sick and infirm.[44] The focus was outward; they created a space for another which prompted this outer response to host the stranger. In practical terms, the brothers created monastery hospitals, taking the sick and infirm into their homes, and into their very lives. The brothers became the host to the stranger. I became intrigued by how hospitality was lived out in such practical and concrete ways. What was it about hospitality that created this interior attitude of receptivity, and how did it become a spiritual practice?

I had the opportunity to explore this question more deeply while I was attending a post-graduate program at the University of St. Louis. One of the requirements for a pastoral counseling and spiritual direction program I attended was to research the charism of the religious institute to which I belonged. Charisms are spiritual gifts, special graces that are freely given by a benevolent God to humankind.[45] We can see how these are shown in the lives of such charismatic leaders like Gandhi, Martin Luther King, St. Francis of Assisi, John of God, and Mother Theresa of Calcutta, to name only a few. In my research for a deeper understanding of the charism of hospitality, I discovered that the actual practice, experience, and reflection of hospitality was the spiritual foundation of the Order to which the brothers belonged. Hospitality wasn't simply about the host adhering to external rules, rituals, or customs, rather, hospitality was both the actual doing of these acts as well as the subsequent reflection on these acts. Every morning, all the brothers, no matter their role, would go to the wards and minister to the patients. This reflection added insight and wisdom which created a spirituality and an interior attitude of hospitality. Not something outside of one's action, but rather, integral to its practice.

Caregivers and Hospitality

Caregivers practice hospitality every day. Their scope of practice requires an openness that allows them to respond to a call at the drop of a hat. They don't have time for a bad hair day or to deal with their personal issues when called to respond to an accident, bank robbery, wildfire, or critical-care patient. Every response demands attentiveness, and every response affects each caregiver differently. This is the first understanding of hospitality of welcoming the stranger. Caregivers, in what is often referred as having people skills, build a report or relationship with those they serve. Showing person interest in the story of the patient or client builds trust and safety. This I call the second understanding of hospitality. Each step takes us deeper into understanding as hosts. Although emotions may temporarily be held in check, eventually they need to be explored and understood. Hospitality is directed toward another and at the same time directed toward the caregiver. In other words, the caregiver must extend the same openness to themselves that they extend to the other. This is the third understanding of hospitality, how the caregiver is affected by their interaction with the patient or client. This is where the one served becomes the healer for the caregiver.

Learning to respond to the needs of others is easy for caregivers; learning to welcome the stirring of emotions of the Soul is more complicated. Not only is the experience of caregiving often missed, but also the opportunity to be supported, fed, and nourished by the very act of caregiving is often neglected. The anthropologist Angeles Arrien argued that the experience of reaching out as a caregiver to one who is ill, in need, or in danger is one of the mysteries of the universe. She suggested the caregiver's experience of responding to one who is ill "is an initiation to coming home again to a deeper sense of self and well-being."[46] Listen to the meaning of Arrien's words—the act of responding, the act of creating space for another, the act of self-sacrificing for another, is a way of finding oneself. Although Arrien focused on the response to illness, I believe a broader understanding can be applied to all acts of caregiving. Wholeness and a renewed understanding of oneself seem to be borne out of the trials and experience of hospitality.

But what is the foundation of this interior attitude, which I believe is a spiritual practice? The act of hospitality is rooted in the interior stirrings of the Soul. It is one thing to believe being a caregiver is my job. It is quite another to believe caregiving is my calling. Years at the bedside as a registered nurse, pastoral counselor, and executive leader would lead me to a deeper understanding of hospitality. Was I willing to be hospitable not only to those I was called to serve, but more importantly, was I willing to become aware of welcoming those interior movements of my Soul?

In the next section, we will explore how the three dimensions of hospitality affected me as I welcomed a new patient into the hospital. Peter and his family taught me to listen not only to him and to his family, but also to my own inner stirrings.

Untangling the Cords that Bind Us

As I prepared to knock on Peter's door, I remembered the words of Dr. Christina Puchalski, a dear friend and colleague: "When you knock on the door of a patient, take a deep breath and know why you are entering the room."[47] Knocking on the door became a reminder for me to stop and create that interior space of welcoming, so I could be receptive to Peter's story. Peter was admitted suffering from pneumonia and inflammation of his lungs—a complication of AIDS which often occurs during its last stages. I was the Catholic chaplain on duty that evening.

After introductions, I asked Peter if I could sit on the chair next to his bed. His eyes welled up with tears as he said to me: "You don't know how long I have waited for someone like you to come and visit me." There was no time to dismiss the compliment, which caregivers often do, or to have visions of grandiosity. I had to understand what he meant. What was Peter really trying to say? As a gay man, Peter was estranged from the Catholic church, yet he still had a deep desire to find reconciliation within his faith and reclaim a sense of belonging.

Peter came from a large Catholic Italian family. He struggled to reconcile his sexuality with his family's beliefs and with Catholic doctrine. Peter also knew he was dying and sought comfort and support. He asked for the sacraments. Tears ran down his face as he discovered a deep peace; he was grateful someone understood. This was important, not only because it alleviated his feelings of isolation, but also because he and his partner were coping with their decision not to inform Peter's parents that he was sick or in the hospital. I knew I would have to explore this with him and his parents sooner rather than later. Peter asked if I could help, and I reassured him that I would help in any way I could. I told him I would check on him in the morning, but if he wanted me to come earlier, he could call the hospital operator who would page me. Then, Peter reached out to hug me. We embraced and said good night.

Paged to Go to My Office

As soon as I began my rounds the next day, I was informed that Peter's father, Antonio, was waiting for me in the chaplain's office. He wanted to know if his son was in the hospital. This was the first of three hospitals he intended to visit. Listening to his concerns and fears about his son helped me to understand more about Peter and his father. I understood the importance of confidentiality and the patient's wishes not to let his family know he was in the hospital, and reassured Antonio that I would investigate and get back to him. Soon after, I visited Peter.

"Peter," I said, "your dad was here earlier and wanted to visit you." Peter began to cry and said, "Yes, I do want him to come; I want to tell him what is wrong with me. Can you help me?" Peter expressed his fears and inability to face his family by himself. He had feared confronting them in the past, and now his fears were even more pronounced due to his weakened condition. He couldn't bear the possibility of being rejected. I asked for permission to call his family to come visit and tell them his diagnosis. That afternoon, Peter's dad, Antonio, his mother, Lucia, and two of his brothers, Markus and Georgio, met me in the reception area, and I walked with them to my office.

As I led them down the hall, I felt the intrigue building up. I wanted to be understanding and receptive to the needs of Peter's parents, as they, too, were affected by Peter's illness. They, too, were strangers needing a safe harbor. I had no idea what the outcome of this meeting would be, but I realized its importance. All I could do was to create a space of welcoming and actively and compassionately listen. I shared with them my initial awkwardness in not informing them of Peter's condition until I had his permission.

During our conversation, Antonio asked, "Do you know what is wrong with my son?" There was silence. I waited for some response from one of his brothers with whom Peter had earlier shared his diagnosis, but there was none. Just more silence.

Perhaps the silence was due to their awkwardness in openly discussing AIDS with their parents present. After a couple of minutes (which seemed more like ten), I broke the silence and explained that Peter requested I speak to them on his behalf, as it was too difficult for him. Too many years and opportunities had passed, and the unspoken words weighed heavily on Peter. I told them of the seriousness of his condition: Peter's immune system was failing and his prognosis was poor. You could hear a pin drop, as all were focused on me. I continued, "Antonio and Lucia, your son has AIDS, and he is in the final stages of the disease."

The Sounds of Silence

Surprised and yet not surprised, Peter's mother Lucia tearfully admitted she suspected this was the case all along. Mothers always know. More silence, deliberate silence, as I wanted the silence to permeate their hearts as they searched for answers. They each tried to avoid looking at each other and became more focused on me. I was expecting one of his brothers to speak up and support their parents. Again silence. Then Antonio, looking up sheepishly, his face etched with emotion, asked poignantly, "What should we do?" I paused for a moment, well-aware of the fact that during the height of the AIDS epidemic, many families rejected their gay sons and daughters who were suffering and dying from various complications of HIV. As I made eye contact with Antonio, the words gently came forward from the deepest resources of my heart: "You need to love him!"

Like an arrow aimed at each of their hearts, the truth of what I said allowed them to feel the pain of their son's diagnosis, as well as to see what each of them needed to do. Tears filled the eyes of everyone in room and even I choked up. They all knew that loving Peter was what they both wanted and needed to do. Both Lucia and Antonio seemed to intone at the same time, full of eagerness, full of a parent's love: "Can we see him?" "Yes, of course," I said, "Peter is expecting you."

The nurses on the floor, as well as Peter, knew I was meeting with his family. It seemed the nurses were holding a silent vigil as I escorted the family past the nurses' station and knocked on Peter's door. "Peter," I said, "your parents and brothers want to see you." I vaguely remember what happened next, because I remained outside the room as Lucia and Antonio smothered Peter with hugs and kisses. Then, one by one, Peter's brothers Markus and Georgio took his hand and hugged him. Peter was beside himself, as there was no need for excuses or explanations. There was not a dry eye in the room nor at the nurses' station. Each nurse on duty also came in to meet Peter's family. In a moment, all the worries and fears of a gay son vanished in the embrace, and he experienced nothing but love from his family. We each felt the numinosity of reconciliation, and the silence of the years was finally broken.

It was my privilege to witness their individual fears surrender to a greater collective need to restore the family unity that was such an important a part of their Italian heritage. Peter was no longer a stranger, but a welcomed and restored member of his family. Each day, different members of his family came to visit. When it was time for Peter to transition to hospice care, they came faithfully each day with food and helped his partner with daily care until Peter died three months later. He died happily, reconciled with and surrounded by his large Italian family. The logjam of silence was finally broken in the honesty and the integrity of the love a father has for his son. Peter's illness became a portal for him and his father to begin a needed conversation, one that might have been lost forever if not for this experience.

Conclusion

The ins and outs of hospitality lead one on a journey, a pilgrimage of self-awareness and transformation. Following centuries of tradition and custom across different cultural and spiritual practices, hospitality is ingrained in the Soul of caregivers. While being host to a stranger, the act of hospitality demands an internal discipline to be open, welcoming, and receptive to the stranger who knocks on our door. In a paper for my certification to be a Board-Certified Chaplain for the National Association of Catholic Chaplains, I had to present my personal understanding and pastoral approach to my work as a pastoral counselor.[48] I chose to share my reflections on hospitality which have continued to be a touchstone in my work as a caregiver.

I have come to believe the heart of compassion is hospitality, and the practice of hospitality is the ability to welcome another. To welcome another means to accept and be present to where the other is and to be present to one's pain, abandonment, faith, crisis, doubts, anger, or fears. We can only be present and hospitable to others—as well as empathetic and compassionate—if we remain receptive these same experiences within ourselves. If the caregiver denies their own anger, grief, loss, pain, or suffering, they cannot be hospitable to another.

To be hospitable means to be present in such a way that the dignity of the other is restored through their encounter with the caregiver. Concurrently, as the caregiver welcomes the stranger, they recognize that their own dignity has been restored in the process. This transformation is like the previously mentioned stories of disguised gods or angels who leave their hosts transformed upon their departure. The paradox of this relationship is that the one who wishes to comfort and be a host is also the one who is comforted and transformed. The ins and outs of hospitality define the special relationship each caregiver experiences and is what makes the work we do so rewarding and life-giving.

There is much to develop regarding this interaction between the caregiver, the one in need, and the caregiver's need. There is also much to explore in what some consider to be a minefield of one's emotional intelligence or lack of support or what hinders one in their service to another. This last understanding of hospitality is where the caregiver is faced with their own opportunities of growth, where they meet the sacredness in humanity, and discover their Soul.

A Moment of Reflection

At your own pace, give yourself a moment of leisure to reflect on each question below. Be creative. Reflect with a spouse or friend or trusted coworker. Spend time taking a walk, writing in a journal, writing a poem, tending to a garden, listening to music, writing a song, or drawing a picture.

1. What is one of your favorite stories of being a caregiver that continues to give you goosebumps or makes your eyes water? (I must admit, I was in tears of gratitude as I wrote about Peter and his Family).

2. Can you give an example of when you went out of your way to practice the skill of active listening with one of your clients?

3. In exploring the different dimensions of hospitality, what has been your experience in being the host, in being aware of the client's story, and of recognizing your own feelings?

4. What is most difficult for you in allowing yourself to become aware of what has been most painful for you in your service to others?

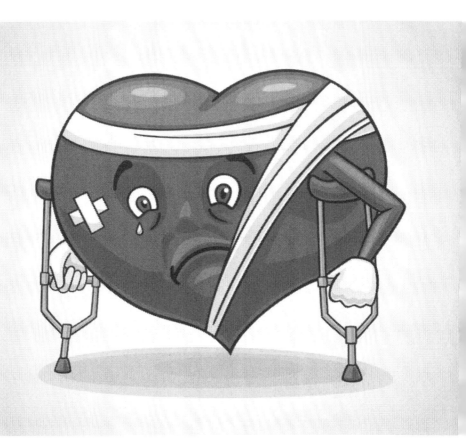

Chapter 6 - Love is a Wounded Healer

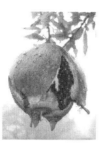

The personal journey of caregivers is a heroic adventure. Heroic, because of all the possibilities of discovering within ourselves our values and strengths, as well as a deeper understanding of woundedness. Woundedness refers to the interior shadow sides of ourselves which seek wholeness and healing. During moments of woundedness, sometimes kicking and screaming, sometimes overcome with the pain of what life has given us, or sometimes lost in the cauldron of heated emotions, we are presented with an opportunity to find meaning. The call, the ability, and the skill to respond to the one in need, to enter a situation that could be fraught with danger, and to be sensitive in responding to woundedness is, I believe, the same ability and skill to enter our own woundedness, which is often revealed in our daily tasks of caregiving.

In a culture that demands perfection in all we do, it is difficult to reconcile that we, as caregivers, skillful and talented as we can be, don't have all the answers. In our daily work, we are confronted with our limitations, personal issues, and woundedness. What within us draws us to the woundedness of others? A skill we often underestimate. Another more poignant question that challenges our imagination and curiosity is: What is it within a person, whether caregiver or the one in need, that draws each to labor with, endure, and come to terms with woundedness, illness, and traumatic events? A mystery not to be solved, but to be explored. This ability to enter, to hold, to guide, and to sustain oneself or another through the mystery of being a caregiver is best understood through the archetypal image of the Wounded Healer.

To say love is a wounded healer is to imply, on the one hand, that caregivers bring their human capacity to care—to be empathetic, to heal, and to create positive outcomes—to every situation. At the same time, caregivers can be confronted with their own limitations, particular boundaries, woundedness, and vulnerabilities that life brings. Herein lies a truth about the paradox of caregiving: a wounded healer responds to one in need, and conversely, the person in need is given the opportunity to be an agent of healing for the caregiver. The very act of caregiving becomes transformational and may lead to the caregiver's personal and professional growth. This may initially appear to be counterintuitive or backward, but it is not.

In Chapter Five, I cited the insight of pastoral counselor William Augsburger who spoke about the unique relationship between caregiver and client.[49] Simply put, when caregivers are sensitive to their own limitations and woundedness, they are better able to understand the woundedness of the one in need and to respond with compassion. This leads to a greater awareness, insight, and growth (for purposes of our discussion, remember we are all caregivers in one way or another).

The archetype of the Wounded Healer conveys the inner reality that within the healer, the person performing the act of caregiving, is woundedness, and within the one wounded, the one seeking care from the caregiver, is a healer. There is a similarity to the Chinese cosmological symbol of the yin and the yang, which acknowledges that within darkness, there is a spark of light, and within the light, there is shadow. The caregiver's sensitivity to the woundedness of the one in need is borne out of self-knowledge and the experience of woundedness. Likewise, the healer function within the one seeking care is activated by the sensitivity and compassion of the caregiver.

Jungian analyst Adolf Guggenbühl-Craig referred to this dynamic as the healer-client function, or what we understand as the caregiver and the one in need. He maintained that when a person seeks a caregiver and healer, an intrapsychic "inner healer" or "healing factor" is also energized.[50]

Who is the Healer: The Caregiver or the One in Need?

This interplay between the caregiver and the one in need is both a humbling and empowering experience. A story from my internship at an outpatient geriatric psychiatric center helps to illustrate some of these dynamics.

During my internship at the psychiatric center, I was asked to facilitate a group session of six to eight clients around the theme of relying on their interior or spiritual strengths to cope with their mental health issues. My intention for the group was to explore whether the clients could discover these pockets of gold within themselves which would help them cope with their illness (I thought this was possible, because I had always believed that a person was more than their presenting diagnosis). We began each session by asking a simple question: "What did you discover about yourself that carried you through the week?"

As holidays approached during the year, memories flooded the room. Each person spoke about how remembering helped them cope with their present and lingering crisis. We had fun to such an extent when one day as I was leaving the group, the attending psychologist asked me, "What do you do in there? They love you." I smiled and said, "We simply support and validate each other." Now, don't get me wrong—we were not holding hands and singing Kumbaya. Yet, we do sing if a client remembers a song, we affirm when someone discovers a way of coping, and we learned to communicate and support each other.

Knowing the time we spent together gave the clients an opportunity to discover more about their coping strengths was in itself a surprising outcome. They rediscovered joy and made a gradual return to the values that shaped their lives and helped them to cope. They were more than their mental health diagnosis. I too shared their joy, the joy of human connection, the joy of being one with them. Within our shared acknowledgement that we are all human and we cope as best we can, our woundedness brought us together in seeking healing and transformation. Roles, titles, and diagnosis gave way to the joy of being one with each other. The energy of the Wounded Healer was present throughout our time together, and in retrospect, I feel they gave me more than I gave to them.

Rediscovering the Spark of Life

One of the members of the group, Shawn, who was admitted for suicidal ideation, asked to see me privately. He was in his early sixties, a World War II veteran who landed on Normandy beach in France. I didn't realize it then, but later learned my father was also there on that December day. Raised in an Irish Catholic family, Shawn grew up impoverished. He wore hand-me-down clothes from his older brothers and the soles of his shoes looked like Swiss cheese. He and his siblings weren't always able to eat, because his parents spent most of the family income on alcohol. Shawn could not wait to leave home and join the army. On the eve of D-Day, being Catholic, he wanted to go to confession, because he realized could be killed. He had a secret to tell the priest, and it took all his courage to say the words, "I'm gay." Shawn expected words of comfort, but the priest simply called him a dog, unfortunately a view held by many religious traditions even to this day I cringed over what Shawn said as the pain he carried seemed like a knife plunged into his heart. And here we were, Shawn and I, sitting in the safety of a sunlit conference room in a Catholic hospital, so unlike that dark and stormy day forty years ago, as the waves of the North Atlantic tossed the ship he was on. Despite his training, Shawn was just a young soldier when he landed on the sandy beaches of Normandy, not knowing if he would live or die. As I gained more insight into Shawn's experiences, thoughts of my father's experience flooded my consciousness

Any of these traumatic experiences could have led Shawn to consider suicide. He was raised in an impoverished alcoholic family whose home seemed like a war zone, and he was gay, which was against the cultural norms of his day. He suffered from symptoms of PTSD from his experience on D-Day until his discharge, and later in the army, was condemned by a Catholic priest. Shawn was challenged in every area of his life, beginning in his home, then in the army, then in a religious context. Being traumatized, rejected, and believing you have no real place in this world could lead anyone to suicidal ideation.

As we focused on his life story, Shawn began to see that even though he had contemplated suicide, he had the inner strength to survive. He was able to make the distinction between wanting to be dead and wanting to end the emotional and psychic pain that was eating at the core of his being. This awareness led Shawn to embrace his real desire to live. His inner strength for survival now gave him the courage to thrive. Shawn was discharged from the program three months later. He tore up his plan for suicide and joined a local support group. I came as the caregiver, yet this group (and Shawn) empowered me as a young intern and encouraged me to continue on as a counselor. I learned that what I was doing was more than a job—it was my calling.

Who is a Wounded Healer?

Who is a wounded healer, and to what extent is the term significant for the caregiver and the one in need? In the broadest sense, we are all wounded healers, as being human guarantees one will experience suffering, limitations, and imperfections. Life has its way, doesn't it? The ancients struggled (as we still do) to understand that a person is not a god, but one whose very mortality signified boundaries, imperfections, and woundedness. There are wounds that are emotional, psychological, and spiritual such as depression, alienation, post-traumatic stress, abuse, and lack of meaning in one's life.

A wound may have many meanings such as a physical cut, a broken bone, a contusion, tumor, or stroke. A wound implies an injury to a living tissue, or the pain experienced by an emotional or psychological injury. Used as a metaphor, woundedness can refer to something as complex as a broken relationship, a loss of reputation, divorce, or loss of employment; in the case of illness, woundedness encompasses a panorama of physical, emotional, psychological, and spiritual experiences. Some wounds may heal, and some may not.

While a wound represents a need to heal, the healer function within a person is an attempt to make us whole.

Jung understood that woundedness is integral to the dynamic processes of self-actualization and individuation. Jung reflected on his personal suffering, search for meaning, and desire to heal, and later, he utilized the insights gleaned from this process of reflection in his psychotherapy practice.[51] Personal growth requires us to acknowledge our weakness, vulnerability, incompleteness, and woundedness, and reflecting on and embracing these very struggles lead to insight, wisdom, and the ability to heal others.

What Does Woundedness Want?

What does woundedness wish to say to the wounded? In the depths of silence, in between the fibers of pain, a voice may be screaming to be heard, unraveling from pain's strong arms.[52] One wound, like the loss of a job due to a company's reorganization, may arouse feelings of anger, disappointment, betrayal, and hurt. On the one hand, these are valid experiences. On the other hand, they may resurface deeper feelings of betrayal, of being left out or even forgotten. The wound cries out for attention and healing, not to be denied, avoided, but to be heard. We caregivers are given the opportunity for self-care by listening to what internally needs to be heard. The wound then becomes a reminder, a voice of a lived experience in the present or in the past. In the words of Dennis Slattery, "wounding is one way the body shows its hyperbole, a way of drawing our attention to it in unexpected ways."[53]

An Unexpected Insight: The Adult Child as Caregiver to a Parent

Annabelle was drawn to woundedness in unexpected ways in becoming the caregiver of her father, who suffered from Alzheimer's disease. Miz Annabelle, as she liked to be called, found that as a caregiver to her father, she discovered something about herself which had been hidden for years. True to her southern heritage, Annabelle excelled in gracious hospitality, manners, and service. Raised in Savannah, her mother taught her the delicate societal norms of being a Southern Belle (after all, her name was

Annabelle!). To say she loved this role is an understatement. She flaunted it anytime she could, often amusing her father, whom she adored. When her mother died two years earlier, Annabelle became the primary caregiver for her father.

In the beginning, the obligation to help became an act of loving service. She had fond memories of their meaningful conversations, but as weeks and months grew into years, her resolve grew thin. "At first," she said, "the feeling of obligation led to spending many hours with my dad." This drew her to experience a deeper understanding of compassion, while at the same time, she noticed her relationship had changed. She was no longer her father's caregiver, but his caretaker. Notice the shift from two adults communicating equally with each other to one of a parent-child relationship, with Annabelle now acting as the parent. Slowly, Annabelle realized her father was slipping more and more away from her, present in the body but no longer present mentally, emotionally, or spiritually.

Annabelle was experiencing the first symptoms of anticipatory grief, which is when one begins to realize something has changed; the person is physically present, yet the real person, the one you know and love, has left the room. Then one day Annabelle's pastor asked her how she was feeling. Annabelle sighed and tried to sort out the emotion she felt. It was like unraveling a string from a ball of yarn felt buried inside her. "I feel numb," she responded. Yes, numb, because she had been burning full throttle on all her cylinders, not realizing she was worn out and had used up all her reserve energy. Numbness implies a loss of energy, a loss of distinguishing one feeling from another because for so long she had to stuff her feelings in deference to her father's needs. Annabelle was beginning to experience the first symptoms of severe compassion fatigue. The feeling that clearly emerged was one of guilt. Was she doing enough?

With her pastor's help, Annabelle started questioning, "Am I selfish if I consider my own needs?" No easy answers emerged, as being overwhelmed clouded her judgment. She was consumed by meeting her father's needs. If she only tried a little harder, spent more time, tried more remedies, would that give her more time with him? Unconsciously, she was trying to fill a bottomless hole, perhaps to protect herself from experiencing the inevitable loss of her father. We caregivers sometimes fail to recognize, just as the ancients did, that we are not gods. The addiction to perfection only becomes self-defeating. The walls of her Southern façade could not protect her. Annabelle pondered. And then she began to question, "Where does selfishness come from? Why would I blame myself or feel guilty about meeting my own needs?" Consider what she discovered in exploring the definition of selfish: inconsiderate, thoughtless, ungenerous, self-indulgent, uncharitable, and self-aggrandizing.[54] Clearly, this was not the case. If anything, Annabelle was selfless, disregarding herself and her own interests. Selfless to such a point that she silenced the inner promptings of her Soul, which encouraged her to care for herself. It is important to note that her father's illness, and the experience of her own lack of self-care, were now her teachers—they had brought her to this place of deep questioning.

Wearing the mask of a Southern Belle taught Annabelle that self-care was only for weak, incapable, or solipsistic individuals (many caregivers fall into this trap). Although Annabelle's relationship with her father had changed, he still became the catalyst that brought down Annabelle's walls of perfectionism, which crumbled like the walls of Jericho. She no longer had to be a steel magnolia as she was experiencing what a wounded healer is. This experience gave her permission, for the first time in her life, to recognize her own vulnerability, her fears, and her limitations, and at the same time allowed her to discover hidden strengths and her capacity for personal growth and transformation.

Each encounter is an opportunity for both the caregiver and the one receiving care to enter a healing relationship. Discovering the healer function within the emptiness of one's woundedness is the dynamic of a wounded healer. Jung called this the process of individuation.[55] Joseph Campbell[56] believed this process is a mystery to be lived, and Hillman referred to this dynamic as "Soul-making."[57]

Common Through the Ages

Within western philosophy, Plato recognized the importance of the physician as a wounded healer. In *The Republic*, he argued that the most skillful physicians are those who have suffered and learned from a variety of illnesses. Rather than being models of good health alone, they became eloquent examples of the wounded healer. He shared his insights about disease and the need for a physician to understand maladies from his own experience. What Plato recognized about physicians can, I believe, be applied to all caregivers.

Essential in understanding the caregiver as a wounded healer is the belief that those who care for others are themselves wounded. This knowledge not only assists them in their care for others, but also allows caregiving to become a personally transformative experience. Woundedness implies that each person has wounds that heal and wounds that are always in the process of healing. Individual and collective memories appear and reappear and become embodied through the remembrance of these stories. Spirit and flesh agonize with crushing pain as memory attempts to bring to light "bit by bit" what needs to be remembered.[58]

An experience of a traumatic event, such as domestic violence, a natural disaster, combat experiences, and physical and sexual abuse may result in wounds that are healed "bit by bit" (such as the recurring symptoms of PTSD). Memories bring us both blessings and wounds, and their constant reappearances call out for recognition and awareness. Storytelling and myth can help caregivers reimagine themselves as wounded healers, which allows them to recontextualize their difficult or even overwhelming memories and experiences within the collective narrative of humanity.

Chiron

In the world of Greek mythology, where the ancients imagined a pantheon of gods in struggling to deal with the mysteries of life, the divine physician Chiron, a centaur and the teacher of the renowned physician Asclepius, is one of the most well-known examples of a wounded healer. The centaurs were creatures with the bodies of horses and with chests, arms, shoulders, and heads of men, who were the descendants of Apollo. Mythos attempted to image the reality of a union between spirit and flesh, reason and instinct, which are components of each person. Animal, human, and divine instincts are combined in the image of the centaur Chiron.

Scholar of religion and mythology Christine Downing commented that Chiron "was wise and gentle," and explained "his animal nature seemed to signify an attunement to instinctual wisdom and a deep understanding of embodiment, an understanding that informed his gifts as hunter, sculptor, and healer."[59] Chiron suffers an incurable wound inflicted upon him by a poisoned arrow from Hercules. Is an incurable wound a metaphor to remind us we are still in a process of becoming? Who among us has reached their full potential as a being human? Sometimes Soul pain reminds us of our desire and longing to continue in our process of growth and transformation, simultaneously recognizing our limitations, needs, and areas of self- improvement.

As caregivers, being wounded is synonymous with being imperfect, with limitations of the being human. Don't you just love the wiggle room this gives us? The fact that Chiron has an incurable wound becomes a metaphor for all of us. In a culture that promotes striving for excellence at a manic pace, it is reassuring to acknowledge what we already intuitively know: no one is totally perfect or complete. Emotional, physical, psychological, and spiritual suffering, which springs forth from the depths of our Soul pain, may lead one to insight and transformation. Simply put, woundedness is a part of being human.

Wisdom Gleaned from Woundedness

The underlying insight of Chiron's incurable wound is that knowledge is gleaned from our wounds. Descent into the liminal space of one's limitations offers both the caregiver and the one in need an opportunity to find meaning in the energies of the wounded healer. Caregiver and the one in need each become a transformative agent for the other. The paradigm of the incurable wound provides a unique perspective about being a wounded healer: our wounds are integral parts of being human. So, when we're hurting, don't understand what we are feeling, or just experience the numbness of being overwhelmed, instead of beating ourselves up, feeling out of control, or feeling afraid of what is buried within, we can begin to accept and learn from the wonderful gift of being human.

Control Vs. Vulnerability

The monster of illness did not overcome Bill as he felt a sudden pain and compression in his chest. He had been working excessively hard to meet some deadlines and assumed what he was feeling had to do with stress. However, the pain did not go away, and the compression became worse. The onset of a possible heart attack brought Bill to a different level of consciousness, albeit reluctantly. Independent and self-reliant, acknowledging a crack in the wall he built around him, Bill admitted he needed help. Giving in to his son's demands, he called 911 and within minutes he was brought to the emergency room. Since he had never been seriously sick before, this excursion was more like going to another planet. Bill was an architect, accustomed to developing plans and meeting deadlines. This date with illness was not penciled in on his calendar.

The emergency room staff recognized the possibility of a major heart attack and quickly surrounded Bill, who bristled at the unwanted attention. "Why all the fuss?" he protested under his breath. Good old Bill, true to form, independent, stubborn, and not allowing anyone, even himself, to experience the fears simmering within. Vital signs, heart monitors, and an intravenous drip with medications were in place. Blood samples, more monitoring, a thousand questions, and more tests followed. If Bill felt steady and calm before he arrived, his anxiety level increased as he was being treated in an emergency room that was unlike any building he had previously designed. To his surprise and delight, all the tests were negative (or so they seemed). Bill decided he should go home. "We want to keep you overnight for observation," the doctor instructed. This was not a part of Bill's agenda. Again, he felt out of control.

Put another way, Bill found it easier to leave than to admit there was the possibility of having a real problem with his heart. Something had to be let go, mainly his resistance to receiving help. He needed to accept his own vulnerability and acknowledge he needed additional medical care. Going home to what was familiar seemed easier than to enter the unknown journey of illness. The doctor looked Bill sternly in the eyes and said, "Yes, you can leave, but I cannot guarantee you will be alive by the time you get out to your son's car in the parking lot." Shaken by the doctor's warning, Bill relented and stayed overnight in the hospital, and in doing so, learned something about self-care. Something within Bill had to metaphorically die so he could live. This was one of Bill's rites of passage.

From Campbell's point of view, these rites of passage are synonymous with the trials of the hero, which "demand a change in the patterns not only of the conscious but also of the unconscious life"[60] How important it is to learn and to be willing to let go. Follow up tests indicated that Bill required open heart surgery to fix three blockages in his heart.

Asclepius

Asclepius, the Roman name for the Greek god of medicine, Asklepios, is as mysterious as the art of medicine itself. Spanning more than 1,000 years of western history, from primordial sagas and heroic tales to a deified mortal and god, again, god representing the search for the sacred, the legend of Asclepius captures the imagination and needs of those who suffer more than any other Greek or Roman god. There is a metamorphosis in the development of the myth of Asclepius. He emerged first in Thessaly, Kos, and Epidaurus where his Asklepios, or temples, were built and became known throughout Greece and later in Rome.

The Oracle of Apollo is at the heart of the healing rituals throughout ancient times. When someone was sick, they did not seek a human clinician alone, but a divine one, since it was believed that illness was caused by the gods and therefore, could only be cured by a god or other divine intervention. Even today, when we are faced with a traumatic event or diagnosed with a serious illness, we ask ourselves, "Is God punishing me?" It was common in the Jewish thought that illness was caused by God or a result of one's sins. Common in early Islamic belief was that only God can heal.[61] Healing becomes a divine and sacred action, and when it is invested with such dignity, caregiving has the inexhaustible advantage that it can be vested with a healing power. This insight is critical in understanding the archetypal energies of the wounded healer because, as C. J. Groesbeck suggested, the wound itself is vested with its own healing power.[62]

Asclepius is one of the only Greek gods who experiences death. His fame, like no other god, prevailed until the third century CE, when many deities faded and were lost. His symbols of a snake and staff continue to be the emblem of modern medicine and healing. Asclepius is divinized as a mortal-god, and even later, during the first centuries of Christianity, he was seen as a prototype of Jesus Christ. Parallels to Asclepius and Christ began to emerge early. Both were born of divine fathers and human mothers. Each was raised by a foster father, Chiron and Joseph. Each suffered, died, and descended into Hades, and each rose and ascended to the heavens. The serpent, a symbol of transformation, became a symbol for each.

Though there are similarities, there is one remarkable difference between the portrayal in art of Asclepius and Christ: Asclepius's curing mission may have resembled that of Christ, but there are no pictures of Asclepius shown in the act of healing. In contrast, there are numerous depictions of Christ performing miraculous cures. He is shown touching those he is curing, such as the leper, the paralytic, and the blind. The miracles of Asclepius were recorded in stone, while those of Christ were illustrated and replicated in tender detail on tombs, reliefs, tableware, and clothing, in addition to the Christian scriptures.[63]

Ancient physicians like Asclepius participated in divine acts of healing. Kerényi suggested it is the physician's awareness of the divinity and sacredness of his healing art "which transplants wisdom into medicine and medicine into wisdom. And the physician who is a lover of wisdom is the equal to a god"[64] Again, god refers to humankind's attempt to understand the sacred or transcendent aspect of the one who cares, the caregiver. Said differently, the energy of our call as caregivers empowers us in developing the skills of our profession. In our acts of hospitality, the mercy and compassion of God inspires us. We are given the opportunity to experience the sacredness of our work, even if only dimly.

Christ: The New Divine Physician

With the rise of Christianity, Christ became the new divine physician, the wounded healer who takes upon himself the woundedness of humankind. He becomes the Suffering Servant of Yahweh (as prefigured in Isaiah 53:5). He is lifted up for all to see (John 3:14) and becomes metaphorically like Asclepius, the divine serpent, a worm and no man, whose image becomes a sign of hope to those who enter into the underworld of darkness, woundedness, illness, and sin. Henri Nouwen described how the mythology of the Wounded Healer is present in Hassidic stories and in the Christian symbolism of the crucifixion, and how the extraordinary healing presence and power of healers was attributed to weakness or woundedness within them.[65]

An Image of Disfigurement

The wounded figure of Christ became more than an image to Katherine, who was rushed to the hospital with internal bleeding. She was visiting friends when she collapsed. At the hospital, an ovarian tumor was discovered, and she was immediately sent to surgery.

During her recuperation, I came to see how Katherine was coping. She talked about the shock of the surgery, the fact that she had a hysterectomy and how she struggled with her own image of being a woman. She felt not only a physical disfigurement, but also an emotional and spiritual one. I listened as Katherine continued: "I know in time, I will heal and understand more fully the mystery of wholeness. At this time, however, I find myself grieving and knowing something that was a part of me is no longer there. I woke up crying during the night and in the empty space I experienced, my eyes caught a glimpse of a crucifix hanging on the wall. A calming voice came over me as words not my own, and yet, so very much my own, echoed through my lips: "You understand. You understand what and how I am feeling. Reflecting on the disfigurement Christ experienced caught me by surprise. I simply do not know what I would have done if I didn't see that crucifix hanging on the wall."

Katherine identified with a disfigured Christ, a god who suffers. She was able to identify her own suffering with that of another whose mutilated body hung before her. Naked, lost in the agony of suffering, and feeling no longer totally human, she felt abandoned, and at times, forsaken. Paraphrasing the words of Psalm 22, Katherine felt less than a woman, maybe like one of the lowliest of creatures, like a worm, no longer human. The psalmist uses the image of a worm to describe this disfigurement: "O my God, I cry by day, but you do not answer; and by night but find no rest. But I am a worm and hardly human, scorned by others and despised by the people (Ps. 22:3, 7).

From the Depths

The worm is a metaphor for one whose body is mangled and disfigured and no longer considered human. Woundedness brings destruction to both body and Soul. Woundedness also gives insight into healing and transformation. A worm crawls in the underworld of the earth bringing destruction in the consumption of waste materials. At the same time, it brings new life with the aeration and fertilization of the soil. This chthonic creature becomes another symbol for the primordial serpent that crawls on the earth and in Hindu mythology is close to its heartbeat. Like the serpent hanging from the staff of Moses in the Hebrew Scriptures, bringing healing to those who look upon it, this Christ-serpent hangs on the wood of the Cross like the ancient Asklepian symbol of healing and transformation.

This icon captures not only the image of a suffering Christ, but attributes to him the title of the servant of Yahweh. This image and title summarize the ancient images that were prefigured in older spiritual traditions. Important aspects of this icon are the association of the staff or rod and the serpent. The staff symbolizes authority and the tree of life, while the serpent is associated with healing and transformation and with Christ hanging on the wood of the Cross. The ancient divine archetype of healing becomes amplified again in the person of Jesus who becomes the worm and no man. Healing is accomplished by gazing upon and recognizing one's woundedness.

This is both the paradox and the mystery that is hidden within this ancient symbol of healing. The symbol becomes the icon of Soul-making, the creative place where beauty is active and reflected. So universal is this symbol that it has become the symbol of modern medicine, the caduceus. The power of the wound awakens the healer function which is sleeping within the afflicted, and it simultaneously activates and supports the caregiver.

An Islamic Perspective

The Qur'an promises good rewards and high rank for those who possess knowledge coupled with faith and practice. According to 13th century Islamic philosopher Al-Faruqi, Islamic science is the practical knowledge that produces results and leads to virtue, the object of the Muslim's prayer: "Oh God grant us a knowledge that is useful and beneficial."[66] The medieval Islamic world produced some of the greatest medical thinkers in history. They made advances in surgery, built hospitals, and welcomed women into the medical profession. Two Islamic physician's lives attest to this.

Al-Razi, The Father of Pediatrics

Abu Bakr Muhammad ibn Zakariya' al-Razi was a Persian physician, chemist, alchemist, philosopher, and scholar who lived in the 9th century. He was a prolific writer, penning over 200 scientific books and articles during his lifetime. As the public became more interested in a scientific view of health, al-Razi searched for causes of illness and possible treatments and cures. Coming out of a belief that only God could cure illness, he integrated his belief with findings from science. He was one of the greatest Islamic medical thinkers in history. Caught in this transition his own insights and sufferings energized him. He wrote:

> The doctor's aim is to do good, even to our enemies, so much more to our friends, and my profession forbids us to do harm to our kindred, as it is instituted for the benefit and welfare of the human race, and God imposed on physicians the oath not to compose mortiferous remedies.[67]

Ibn Sina, Physician and Medical Educator

Ibn Sina (980-1037), whose full name was Abu al-Hussayn ibn Abdullah ibn Sina, was an outstanding medical writer and physician. His *Al-Quanun fi al-Tibb* was a masterpiece of Arabic systemization which incorporated all known medical knowledge. When the work was translated into Latin, it became known as the *Canon of Medicine* and was the dominant text for the teaching of medicine in Europe. He summarized Hippocrates (460-377 BCE), Galen (130-200 CE), Dioscorides (40-90 CE), and late-Alexandrian physicians, adding Syro-Arab and Indo-Persian knowledge along with his own notes and observations. A physician ahead of his time, he was often misunderstood, which led him to more research and study.[68]

Ibn Sina's *Canon of Medicine* was used as a medical text for over 800 years, and its use was continued in some areas until well into the 19th century. It is one of the most famous and influential books in the history of medicine. Ibn Sina's *Canon of Medicine* set standards in the Middle East and Europe, and it provided the basis of a form of traditional medicine. UCLA and Yale University continue to teach some principles of *The Canon of Medicine* in their history of medicine courses.[69] Ibn Sina was a scholar not only in medicine but in law, mathematics, physics, and philosophy. The name Avicenna, as he was known in Europe, is a Latinized form of his Arabic name.

The Prophet Muhammad (PBUH)

Muhammad's (PBUH) willingness to follow the stirrings of his heart led him to enter the darkness of a cave. Like other prophets before him, Muhammad's asceticism and devotion opened his heart and allowed him to listen to God's word. Muhammad's (PBUH) hearing and transmitting the merciful and compassionate Word of God calls to mind other spiritual traditions that were born from insights derived from a struggle with darkness: like Siddhartha who became the Buddha, Moses who climbed a mountain to listen to God in the darkness of the clouds, or Jesus's journey into the wilderness for forty days and nights. As Muhammad (PBUH) wrestled with the angel Gabriel, the words of God began to flow from his lips, a process of struggling and listening. These revelations would later be codified in the sacred writings called the Holy Qu'ran, the Islamic scripture. One of the pillars of Islam, the Month of Ramadan, commemorates Muhammad's annual pilgrimage and asceticism during his prayer and fasting in the cave.

The message of Unity and Union, and the integration of the will of God in one's entire activities, are goals to be admired and pursued. This is the life of a mystic, which I found at the heart of Islamic spirituality. Understanding the *ummah*, a core of Islamic belief, is another surprise and, yes, a challenge. I wonder if it relates to a larger religious question: Is it possible for humankind to have a perfect society? Or is the challenge one of working towards building one? When is one's truth the only truth among many truths in a pluralistic society? Can a unity of beliefs, as envisioned by Muhammad over fourteen hundred years ago, be realized? This is the discipline of Islam.

The Arafah Family

The family of Mrs. Arafah, all devout Muslims, asked to take their deceased mother home from the hospital. Being the administrator on call, the evening supervisor called me for some support. "Can you ask the family why they want to take their mother home," I asked. The supervisor responded, "It was because they wanted to do the ritual washing and felt it could not be done in the hospital." We developed a simple plan to meet the needs of Mrs. Arafah's family. The supervisor told the family that a private room was being prepared where Mrs. Arafah would be transferred from the ICU. There they would have the privacy and the means to do their ritual washings. The mortician would be called when they finished their ritual washings. Family, nurses, and staff contributed to the hospital event as a collective experience of wounded healers.

Parzival's Quest as a Wounded Healer

"What's in a name?" Juliet asks Romeo in William Shakespeare's *Romeo and Juliet*. A name identifies and is linked to cultural and mythological stories that often reveal a hidden meaning or a special identity. The name Isabel, for example, means one who is pledged to God, while the name Edward connotes a guardian or protector of riches. Interesting, then, is the 12th century German story of Parzival, whose name means "pierced through the heart."[70] Piercing implies a woundedness which may be emotional, psychological, spiritual, and physical. Piercing involves suffering while learning what the call to adventure entails.

Parzival is given a clue about his heroic journey, one in which his suffering will assist him in overcoming his arrogance and pride while moving toward an interior attitude of humility and compassion. Only then will Parzival be able to understand the Grail question and become the Grail King. Being pierced through the heart is another image for being a wounded healer, as Parzival reflects on his own wound as well as the incurable wound of the Grail King, Anfortas.

Heart Intelligence

As discussed earlier, prior to the late 17th century, the human heart was considered the center of a person and the core of imagination. As the symbolic unity of intellect, feelings, and intuition, the heart was the agent of circulation in ancient Greece, the Hindu seat of Brahma, the Islamic throne of God, and the Christian kingdom of God, where the pilgrim travels in the primordial state where God dwells.[71] Parzival represents a different image: a heart that suffers, a heart linked to the earthly endeavors of life.

After Harvey began performing autopsies, the heart became a pump, a technological image; this change signaled a movement from mythos to logos. When the heart becomes purely mechanical, the idea of the sacred mystery is lost. Hillman argued, "How can all that the heart symbolizes such as the courage to live, the center of one's strength and passion, love, feelings, the locus of one's Soul, and identity, how can all this be held in the hands of the physician or the coroner?"[72]

There is a physicality in the beat of the heart, a sense of being embodied and grounded. Listen to the tapping of orchestrated fingers against stretched animal skins synchronizing with the heartbeat of the earth. Ancient music comes alive, stirring the depths of one's Soul. The beat of the heart reminds us of how the heart circulates the integrated life of nature, humankind, and the cosmos. This "heart intelligence" comes alive when there is a simultaneous knowing and loving by means of imagining.[73] In *The Divine Comedy,* the pilgrimage of Dante, guided by Virgil and motivated by the love of Beatrice, is such an example of a simultaneous knowing and loving. Knowing and loving, logos and mythos, create images that give life and inspire. At this juncture of reflection, one experiences enchantment. Campbell called this process aesthetic arrest, which is "that enchantment of the heart by which the mind is arrested and raised above desire and loathing in the luminous stasis of aesthetic pleasure"[74] Part of the power of symbols and myths is that they enchant those who are willing to engage them.

Let's focus again on the original call of the caregiver whose response to the one in need demands a focus and skill to be immersed in the situation at hand. This focus is grounded in compassion, the ground of true morality, as we participate first in responding to the pain of the other, and then in the alleviation of that pain.[75]

This was the case when I responded to an urgent page. Louisa, a daughter whose mother was dying, called for the chaplain. As she held vigil with her mother, she was overwhelmed by conflicting feelings and asked for support and guidance. I knew a compassionate presence was important. However, the loss and grief Louisa felt over her dying mother brought to light a deeper loss she had experienced as a child. "I am so angry at my mother I want to kill her," she sobbed. Talk about the need for direct questions and more active listening! Louisa then told the story of her mother's brother molesting her when she was 10 years old. More compassion, and more listening. "She's dying now. Little good that would do!" Louisa moaned, "Why didn't she believe me? Why didn't she protect me?"

Feelings of rage, sadness, and guilt brought Louisa to the stark realization of the depth of the loss she was now experiencing. She had lost her mother's protection many years ago, and her mother's impending death ignited a long-smoldering flame. In these moments of listening, I knew the process of recovery would be longer than the time I had with Louisa. The beginning of the end began that evening in the compassion I felt; I realized that although the unraveling of her complex grieving would take longer, what was important was the presence I could offer Louisa. Her uncle had died, and she was already seeing a counselor. What she needed now was a validation that her feelings were appropriate.

The journey to healing was indeed complex as daughter and mother now faced each other with only moments remaining to possibly begin a process of forgiveness. Despite her conflicting emotions and feelings towards her mother, Louisa was able to show her love, holding her hand until she died. Holding these conflicting emotions of Louisa, as well as creating the space for her to discover and respond to the different levels of grief she was experiencing, was both a challenge and seasoned skill for me.

John Ciudad: Wounded for Others

Being wounded, literally and metaphorically, is a part of being human. What drew me to the life of John Ciudad was his ability to be comfortable with his own vulnerability, limitations, and woundedness. While the word archetype would have been foreign to John, he had an uncanny ability to reach out to the sick and abandoned individuals living on the streets of 16th century Granada, Spain. Although it is evident John had compassion for those in need and helped them in concrete ways, I also believe he consciously accepted his own struggles, suffering, and limitations. In other words, I think he intuitively understood the universal energies of a wounded healer.

The turning point in John's life occurred during an evening service at a local church. A sermon by the renowned Spanish preacher John of Avila sent John into the streets crying for mercy and forgiveness, overwhelmed by the experience of God's love. Spit upon, bullied, and roughly handled, he tore at his clothes and rolled on the ground; he appeared to be mad. Friends took him to the Royal Hospital where he was shackled and placed in the psychiatric ward. As he regained his strength and insight, he was allowed to help others at the hospital. As mercy was shown to him, he began to reach out to other inmates.

Once released from the hospital, John started a hospice to take in the poor, abandoned, undesirables of the city. He went around the city begging for alms to support his work and said, "Do good to yourselves by doing good to others." It wasn't until I revised this book that his words really hit me. His insight is so direct and yet so profound. Imagine the work and service we caregivers do for others is the source of our transformation, of our salvation! Remember our conversation earlier, when I asked a group of caregivers asking if they felt they became better people because of their service to others. They all nodded their heads in agreement. John Ciudad's words are profound, and his message is still relevant for us.

As his charitable works grew, so did his reputation. He was thought to be either of God or mad.[76] The ancient, universal, and archetypal energies of the wounded healer, of angels and gods appearing when offered hospitality, came alive for John with those who suffered. As the wounded Christ became a model of compassion to John, he strove to become a model to those who suffered and were ill.

Two events reveal how John's practice of hospitality entertained gods and angels. On the first occasion, John came across a wounded beggar lying in the streets. He attempted to pick him up and carry him to his hospice, but at first, he could not lift him. Finally, he tried again and found he was able. He realized he was being assisted by the archangel Raphael, whose name means "God heals." This scene was captured in a painting by the 16th century artist Bartolome Murillo, who attempted to portray how divine energies and strengths assist us. In a moment of weakness, John found the interior archetypal strength and grace to care.

On another occasion, John was washing the feet of one of the residents in the hospice. As he continued to wash, John noticed wounds on the resident's feet. He looked up and realized he was washing the feet of Christ. The one who was wounded became a healer to the one washing his feet. Whether Christ literally appeared or not, the insight John experienced was a reminder of the sacredness of his work. Angels and gods did appear. What is inspiring to me as a caregiver, and as a former member of the Hospitaller Brothers of St. John of God, is that John, while being locked up in a mental institution, in one of his darkest moments, discovered his call to service. Why do we fear being vulnerable, when in reality, within our vulnerability, we may discover our strengths?

The following story captures the experience of James who, in discovering the ramifications of a diagnosis of myeloma, was thrust into a strange and unfamiliar world. At the core of his being, he struggled with the tension of experiencing his need for help while remaining in charge as best he could.

Drifting Out to Sea, Yet Moored by Family

The complexity of both the medical center and his diagnosis led James into a dark place of uncertainty. Unanswered questions moved him beyond impatience to a mild state of fear and anxiety as he lay in his hospital bed. The currents of the day, such as his tests being postponed, the doctors not showing up, the idleness of what appeared to wasted time and not getting things done efficiently, sent James adrift in an unknown sea. Dealing with a new diagnosis of cancer was difficult enough but waiting to learn to its extent and possible treatments seemed more unnerving than the actual diagnosis. "Mark," James remarked to his nurse, "I feel like I have drifted out to sea, without a compass, without knowing which direction to go." James found an image to convey what he found difficult to express, his own lack of control, ambiguity, and vulnerability.

The tidal wave of uncertainty that surrounded him sent him to an unfamiliar place, a place where he experienced doubt and uncertainty. Within this liminal space of "betwixt and between," James waited, drifting, and numb to the possibility of finding a compass hidden within him. Insight gradually came as he became conscious of his wife, Amy, sitting beside him holding his hand. His daughter, Carol, a research analyst for a drug company doing trials for cancer patients, already had arranged a consultation with the leading cancer expert on myeloma in the state. His son, Scott, who worked out of state, was arriving the next weekend to assist with chores around the house. Simultaneously, James found himself drifting and yet being moored by the lifeline his wife, son and daughter were providing. This new world of liminality was messy, uncertain, and unnerving. A threshold of affliction had been crossed. A threshold that caregivers often face when we find ourselves drifting into uncharted situations. Along with the professional caregivers providing care for James, his wife and his children also joined the caregiving team.

Swept Across the Threshold

Illness is a threshold that we cross involuntarily, as if we're caught in a receding tide. James's experience of drifting out to sea is such an example. The threshold he crossed separated him from the world he knew as he entered the hospital. The doors of the medical center might be likened to the jaws of a whale that seemed to swallow him into the darkness of both his inner world and the world of the medical establishment, like Jonah descending into the underworld in finding himself in the belly of a whale (Jonah 1:17). Without understanding the implications of this passage, James passed through the liminal jaws, the permeable wall, and the artificial barrier we impose between myth and reality.[77] Questions such as what is real or imagined arise. Like the curtain separating one hospital bed from another, this questioning restrains yet captures the realities on both sides of the curtain. The permeable partition that the curtain signifies holds the tension of opposites between what is a myth and what is reality.

Within his angst, James found an image to express an experience that was unknown to him, the image of drifting out to sea. While this image expresses movement, the image of drifting also became an image that grounded James in the reality of his experience as a person with cancer. Some things were beginning to change. James was totally unaware that he too would be changing in this process. The "James" he had known was beginning to experience a metamorphosis: self and ego were in the process of dying and being renewed.

Relevance for Today

In 1951, Jung first used the term "wounded healer." Reflecting on his life experience, he came to believe that in any ongoing doctor-patient relationship, the whole personality of both patient and doctor is called into play. While he specifically referred to the time-honored doctor-patient relationship, we, as caregivers, can apply the same understanding to ourselves. Jung wrote "the doctor is effective only when he himself is affected . . . only the wounded physician heals. But when the doctor wears his personality like a coat of armor, he has no effect."[78] For a moment, reflect on the difference between just "doing your job" versus the deeper call that motivates you as a caregiver.

Common Usage

Psychologist Len Sperry observed that the term "wounded healer" has recently been used synonymously with burnout or impairment of caregivers in the healing professions.[79] He recognized the term is not new and has been associated with a sacred tradition across several cultures throughout the ages. The relationship between woundedness and healing is a truth recognized in myths and rituals of traditional cultures throughout the world. Serge Daneault questioned whether this archetype could assist physicians. For Daneault, the wounded healer is a person who has become a source of great wisdom, healing, and inspiration precisely because of the suffering they have endured.[80]

The physician becomes a healer as his technical skills are guided by his experiences and self-reflection. Dr. Martin Lipp added: "My wounds become my spectacles, helping me to see what I encounter with empathy and a grateful sense of privilege"[81] The patient facilitates the doctor's own healing by discovering the interior resources that allow healing and transformation to occur. Each is involved in a process that activates a healer function from within. Finding Soul invites the wound to speak, holding and listening tenderly and compassionately to the promptings from within.

Conclusion

The psychic energies of the Wounded Healer contain the ability for both the caregiver and for the one being served to hold what seems impossible to be held. The healer must first recognize their own wounds to make space and understand the woundedness of the other. So necessary is this inner work of the caregiver that without it there is a danger healing may not occur, not only for the one in need but also for the caregiver. An understanding of one's personal woundedness, suffering, and illness appears to be a prerequisite for the caregiver and for the one in need.

Empathy and compassion are drawn from these experiences, because, as Downing suggested, an awareness of woundedness "is a prerequisite for taking on the role of healer."[82] The miracle of participating in the archetypal energies of the Wounded Healer is that the one who suffers discovers the capacity for and the possibility of healing and of one's human dignity being restored through the encounter with the caregiver. Concurrently, in facilitating this process, the caregiver rediscovers his or her dignity being restored and renewed. Face to face with life, the caregiver is challenged to find meaning in the mystery of caregiving. There is an interchange between the caregiver as host and the client as a stranger in need. Creating interior space to receive the stranger is an interior act of the Soul. So, too, is creating the time, energy, and space for caregivers to understand their experiences.

A Moment of Reflection

1. Was there a particular insight or question that emerged during your reading of this chapter?

2. Do you relate to being a wounded healer?

3. What, in your service to others, excites you and gives you joy?

4. What animates and sustains you in your profession?

5. Are you conscious of your strengths that support and nourish you?

_____

_____

_____

_____

_____

_____

_____

_____

_____

_____

_____

_____

_____

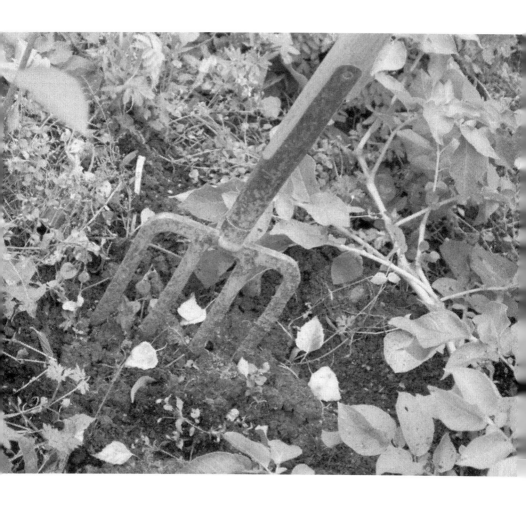

Chapter 7 - Tending the Soul's Garden: Reclaiming the Art of Reflection

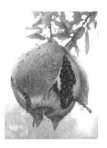

This chapter addresses a skill we all have as caregivers: the ability to reflect. We do it all the time in our professional and personal lives. We plan, explore options, and execute them. All are opportunities for reflection. Each project, each experience, each job well done can lead one to pause and ponder. These reflections may lead one to change a procedure or a policy, or to make future decisions. Change is what occurs outside oneself, but tending to the Soul's garden implies an interior change, perhaps even a transformation.

Author and speaker William Bridges argued that, culturally, we often confuse the two. Change is situational, like deciding to develop a new skill, move the furniture around, paint your office a different color, or accept a promotion. Transformation, on the other hand, is about interior change, about listening to one's Soul, about learning from experience, commonly called a change of heart. It is not a static event but one that is dynamic and implies movement. Transformation is being on a hero's journey where one gains insight and a psychological awareness about one's inner reorientation and self-redefinition which needs to occur for the change to work.[83]

It is worth noting that Bridges's understanding of the process of transformation is similar to the hero's journey as outlined by Joseph Campbell. The hero's journey consists of a call, a leave-taking where one descends into the netherworld where the hero faces trials, uncertainties, monsters, and chaos. The journey challenges the hero or heroine to win the boon or the prize, to achieve a new status, and to make a victorious return.

Like Campbell, Bridges realizes the process of transformation is dynamic. The first phase of this process often begins with an ending—a phase of life, or a life event occurs that marks the end of a circumstance, be it personal or professional, positive or negative. For example, receiving a promotion or an inheritance, experiencing the birth of a child, or leaving home to attend college could each signify endings that initiate the process of transformation. Other examples include the death of a family member, the end of a marriage, losing a job, or experiencing a natural disaster such as a flood, hurricane, or wildfire. Each of these events leads the individual into phase two, a period of uncertainty, distress, and chaos. The death of a family member leads one into a new world that no longer includes them. The ending of a marriage leaves one with the uncertainty of the future, as does being made redundant at work. Traumatic events challenge one's interior belief systems as something has radically changed such as one's safety. Finally, the journey may lead one to the third phase of transformation which is a new beginning, such as a new job, a new experience, a new freedom, and a new awareness of one's interior strengths. In summary, there is an ending, a wondering, and a concluding with a new beginning.[84]

An Innate Skill

Caregivers face these experiences day in and day out as life continually teaches them the pains and joys of being human. One cannot remain neutral, as caregiving has its way of transforming the caregiver. Each event, each act of service, each encounter with the one being served has an impact on the caregiver. Most of the time, the experience leads the caregiver to a greater appreciation of who they are as caregivers. Sometimes, the caregiver partakes in traumatic events which may take more time to debrief and may require time for self-care. Sometimes, the experience of these traumatic events leads to the caregiver experiencing different symptoms of compassion fatigue, which leads to burnout or secondary stress disorder.

Who doesn't appreciate a job well done, knowing you've given yourself so selflessly in the work you do? How about your experience of savoring or lingering over a glass of red wine after a homemade pasta dish? These moments are borne out of our experiences, the wonderful events in our lives. Yet each of these experiences may also be transformative, the acceptance of appreciation may lead one to a greater work ethic and lingering over a glass of wine may lead one to greater insight and the experience of gratitude. The skills we have learned as caregivers were not taught in a vacuum but developed and improved by reflecting on our experiences. It is how we learn. It is also how our lives can be transformed.

For a moment, reflect on your career. Can you remember how you first felt as a student nurse or teacher, a new member of the emergency medical team (EMT), your experience as a first responder, or a physician intern, still wet behind the ears, compared to how you feel now? There was a call to service, a new beginning, and then delving into the work, a wondering and an exploration, along with many challenges, mistakes, and trials. I remember as a student nurse having difficulty with a particular patient. Yes, I know now, I was challenged to learn from this experience. I remember discussing this with my student advisor and she said, "Ed you will learn from this, but you don't have to like every patient." That was a relief. I also had difference experiences of achievement, a new beginning, an arrival at the accomplishment, of certitude, learned wisdom, and growth. Insights gained from our experiences have made us better caregivers. This is the miracle of caregiving. We, who seek to heal, the wounded healers, are transformed in the act of healing. Without any promptings or manuals, we were taught the process of reflection. Reflection is the tool that cultivates the garden of our Soul; by tending to the emerging memories and images, a history of who we are is revealed.

In the next section, I tell the story of one of my first experiences as a graduate nurse. Maestro! A little music, it is time for a moment of reverie.

A Lighthearted Lesson

One of my most light-hearted experiences as a graduate nurse was when I was assisting a physician intern at the bedside of a patient named David. David's gastric feeding tube needed to be replaced. Simple. We discussed the procedure with him as we prepared the treatment table. The doctor then cut the stitch holding the tube in place, and the tube was easily removed. As we were getting ready to insert a new one, turning towards the treatment table, David decided to let us know he was still in charge despite his recent suffering a stroke which affected his gag reflex. He decided to cover the stoma or opening, with his arm. When we turned ready to insert the tube, the patient expanded his belly, so the indentation of his belly button appeared to be the stoma. In a flash, we knew this was not the intended opening. Almost instantly the patient began to laugh and picked up his arm. I think I chuckled more than the intern as we realized there was a vast difference between a surgical stoma and the depression of his belly button. We both learned not to take things too seriously, as the David provided a bit of comic relief for each of us. From the storeroom of your life, can you retrieve and bring forth experiences that bring a smile to your face? Reflection allows us to glean insights from our experiences which help us gain perspective and balance in our acts of caregiving.

The Caregiver as Active Participant

Consider for a moment the different insights you've experienced in reading the preceding chapters. Do you remember our discussion in Chapter One about reflection being a process of stepping back and reviewing one's experience and memories of an event? Sometimes stepping back recalls pleasant, even joyful experiences. Other times, we may be confronted with personal and professional experiences which are sad, even painful. Our Soul has a way of bringing up issues and memories that need healing.

As such, the caregiver is often engaged on many different levels. On one level, the caregiver may act as a skilled tactician, while on another level, they are relationally involved with the client; finally, they are engaged in an exploration of their experience of the event. Let me give you an example of such an experience when I was the participant, almost like in a Greek Tragedy, actively listening to the one affected, and then realizing I needed time to explore what was happening within me because of this experience. The call to visit a patient, the descent into the experience of the patient's mother, and the outcome, a new understanding about self-care.

Personal Suffering Masks as Anger

When I knocked on the door, I thought this would be a routine visit welcoming a new patient to the rehabilitation unit. I was greeted by the mother of the patient, Mrs. Morales, who immediately recognized me from our encounter three weeks ago when her daughter, Angela, was admitted to the intensive care unit. Before I could even introduce myself, she asked, "Do you remember me?" I immediately recalled the patient care conference, when the neurosurgeon called to discuss Angela's treatment options, as she was suffering from a cerebral hemorrhage. As we discussed the meeting and the outcome of the conference, something triggered Mrs. Morales to engage in an outburst of anger at the neurosurgeon. She was furious, even vitriolic. I just listened, realizing it was not about me, a trap many caregivers find themselves in when confronted with anger. I surmised Mrs. Morales's anger and frustration were a cover, most likely for the deep pain she was feeling over her daughter's diagnosis—Angela was paralyzed at the age of thirty-four. As a pastoral counsellor, I imagine she trusted me enough to vent her frustration, giving her permission to cry out, even to God.

My intuition told me to simply listen to Mrs. Morales, because her anger was authentic and needed a voice. As children and as adults, few of us were rewarded for expressing anger. Granted, there are appropriate ways to express our anger, but dammit, the first step is to admit we are angry; the second step is to express it appropriately.

No one I know likes to be the scapegoat for another person's anger. Likewise, the person expressing their anger is responsible for understanding its root causes, and it is up to them to find an adequate way to express it. I knew, given the allotted time, the best I could do was to listen. Not everything would be taken care of in one pastoral visit. Nor did it have to be. It was enough that she could voice her real feelings which most likely had been brewing ever since her daughter's accident, I just happened to be the person at the right time for the eruption to occur (Lucky me, I thought). However, caregivers often blame themselves for the angry outbursts of others, when indeed it has nothing to do with them. I don't know what I said to Mrs. Morales or how I left the room, I just remember walking down the hall (which seemed longer than usual), leaving the rehabilitation unit, and entering the hospital. Then, something within me compelled me to speak with one of my colleagues on the fifth floor.

As I walked out of the elevator, before I even had the chance to speak, Susanne smiled at me. When I came more into view, her smile turned to concern, then to alarm. "Ed," Susanne remarked, "You look terrible. What happened?" I remember distinctly putting my hands together over my head and, as if holding a trowel, I began making hand-scraping movements and told Susanne I must scrape all the anger off me. I actually said, "Susanne, give me a moment to scrap all this shit off of me, it is not about me."

That day, I learned caregivers often become the target or scapegoat for clients or their family members to vent. I learned many lessons that afternoon, such as active listening, presence, and the realization that I did not have to fix anything. The question was whether I was willing to do the interior work to further explore the lessons. Was I hospitable enough to welcome one who masquerades her Soul pain with anger? I knew I had to welcome the client where she was, even if I had to navigate through the sludge of her angry feelings.

Trusting Your Insights

Although I was an active participant in the example above, my role was to welcome the new patient to the hospital and complete a spiritual care assessment. Unable to speak, I still remember the perplexed expression on Angela's face during the exchange. I also became involved with and experienced the trauma of the patient's mother. I knew intuitively her anger was not about me. That insight about not blaming myself was not instant but developed over time, and even as I write this, reflecting on my experience leads me to more insight and discovery. For example, why did she feel safe enough to vent her frustrations with me? Was she crying out to God, who I, as a pastoral counsellor, informally represented? Reflecting on experiences can help us develop increased awareness, insight, and wisdom.

There is a scene in the movie "Children of a Lesser God" that reveals this societal tension of expressing anger. Sarah Norman struggles to express her anger, an anger she has stuffed over the years about being deaf and the rejection she experienced by her father. She reaches the boiling point when she is encouraged to move out of her comfort zone by James, a professor at the school. Desperate and confused about not knowing how to sort out her anger, and simultaneously falling in love with James, Sarah runs away to her estranged mother, only to be followed by James. When he asks why she left him, Sarah says, "I thought that if I faced the anger raging within me, it would kill me. Instead, I learned I am more than my anger and I can face it."[85]

Reflection is at the Heart of Being Human

Did you find yourself daydreaming and gaining insight as you listened to the frustrations and anger of a devoted mother in the preceding story? Were there stories in the earlier chapters which mirrored something about yourself? Did you discover an event that radically influenced you or, in retrospect, may have even been transformative? There may have been something in your life that ended, something that led you to explore a new beginning. My point is this: reflection is at the heart of being human. We do it all the time. It is not a skill reserved for monks, nuns, or mystics in monasteries alone, but an interior process that we as humankind possess, and like everything else we do, we need to practice it. "It is the spark within us," suggested Thomas Merton, "that ignites our intuition and flourishes most purely right in the middle of the ordinary."[86]

Images, then Words

During one of my pastoral counseling classes the instructor asked the class to choose an image that represented an area of personal growth. I began to question the question: "Why an image?" I wondered.

Many images appear in our consciousness. They can be images of joy, like the moment you first met your partner, or images of revery, perhaps a memory of clasped hands, kneeling in front of a candle before a favorite icon or sacred object. Images of fear may emerge, like memories and fragments of traumatic events that, like the tip of an iceberg, reveal hidden and painful emotions. Reflection allows images to emerge. These are not external images, like the pictures we see in magazines, on television, or on the internet. These are interior images that emerge from memories and experiences.

A few years ago, I started a diet. Even before I began, an image of "skinny me" appeared. I loved skinny me. I was filled with joy and remembered when I could turn my body sideways, and you couldn't see me. Before my metabolism changed, I was tall and thin. Then, I started to grow east and west instead of north and south. I envisioned myself going on a spending spree since I was already down a few sizes. These images already had their own stories even before I could express them in words or develop a plan of action. The imagination manifests itself in a variety of ways, and in this instance, the diet elicited the image of skinny me, along with a feeling of yearning to be skinny me again. But the image appeared first, and the words came second.

Earlier, we discussed how imagination comes into play in our daily lives and how it expresses psychic life. According to the Ulanovs, imagination "speaks first in images before it speaks in words."[87] How often do we get tongue-tied trying to articulate an experience that is primarily symbolized rather than verbalized? Somehow, we must listen to what the image wants to say to us, which means we must also create an attitude of listening. Not that this is foreign to us, but like a muscle, we need to exercise and train it. This was the task at hand presented by the professor. Find an image and allow it to speak, as it has a language of its own which leads one to meditation and reflection.

The second part of the exercise was to ask the class if they would support me with the goals I set. Like most caregivers, I was often too busy to stop and reflect on an area of growth or improvement, let alone openly discuss it with my peers (sound familiar?). There was some comfort, however, in knowing that each member of the class was also charged with the same task. We were given about ten minutes to sit in silence and be attentive to what images came to mind. I could already hear the moans and groans of each member in the room, as sitting in silence was not a practice that most of us were familiar or comfortable with. I was also in a transition in my career—some things needed to be changed, while other new beginnings, though exciting, also presented their own unique challenge (again, the call, the journey, and then a new beginning). Although I was initially fearful at the prospect of all these new changes, I knew maintaining the status quo was not an option.

Sprinkle Fertilizer Around Its Roots

As we sat in silence, I realized that, somehow, the ground had been prepared: an image of a peach tree came to light. It was cut back a bit, yet there were new shoots developing around the base of the tree, promises of more fruit. A voice within seemed to say, "Not to worry, just dig around its roots, add a little fertilizer, and all will be well." Dreams of eating those ripened peaches, both sweet and tart, slipped into the numinous realm of my consciousness. The image of the fruit tree led to other images of new shoots and ripened peaches, of the tilled ground, and lastly the star of the kaleidoscope, fertilizer.

Imagine that—fertilizer! But how did fertilizer correlate with my personal growth? "First things first," I mused, "Let's explore what fertilizer actually does." Fertilizer, as you know, has a challenging aroma, yet it provides nutrients necessary for plants, trees, and crops to grow. So, I needed some metaphorical fertilizer. But then what? (I didn't believe the solution involved rolling around on a dung heap.) There was no time to take a deep breath, as the farmer within instinctively knew what *not* to do. I had clear recollections of using it in my garden, as well as almost gasping for air as I drove along California's central coast, past the meandering fields prepared for the planting of lettuce, broccoli, spinach, cauliflower, tomatoes and cabbage.

My mind raced. I knew the next step was to share this image with all thirty members of my class. Was this the only meaning of fertilizer? How could I translate this in a practical way? Was the fertilizer I needed something like developing new goals, spending more time on self-care, understanding my own interior values and processes, or listening more attentively to the inner promptings of my Soul? Somehow, the restlessness within me vanished. I was on to something and wanted to go deeper. My internal dialogue, however, was silenced when I heard my name called. It was now my turn to share the fruits of my musings with my classmates.

As I told the story of a fruitless tree and how it reminded me of a passage in the Christian Scriptures, there was an irony about my words.[88] Then there was silence, a pregnant pause. I looked around the room stumbling to get the words out after the story I just related. Then I said: "Each of you, my classmates, are the fertilizer I need to spread around my roots. Now don't take this literally. The fertilizer is just a metaphor. The image is telling me I need nutrients from a variety of resources, including you, to support, challenge, and cajole me during this coming year." I smiled and looked around the room—my classmates were smiling, too. I knew then that this image was telling me to tend the garden of my Soul.

There weren't any gasps, but a sincere understanding, even a few laughs. Any type of personal growth involves two factors, the personal and the collective. Although there is an individual aspect to growth, something that one holds very close to oneself, any reflective process is enhanced by the support of another, be they a spouse, friend, pastor, or counselor. Caregivers may experience the desire to reflect on a particular event in solitude, because it is often difficult for them to reflect in the company of their colleagues. (Remember Allison's comment earlier that many first responders refer to critical access debriefing as "the crybabies club"). Where did we learn that we have to "tough it out" by ourselves?

Tending to our Soul's garden is an ongoing task requiring attentiveness, careful listening, patience, and the ability to courageously reach out.

The Reflection Urge

It is in the midst our ordinary lives that insights emerge and lead us to moments of reverie and reflection. Reflection is a spontaneous experience, as if we're caught up and lost in the moment, a sort of "time out" which takes us to realms of wonder and excitement, or to places of fear and painful memories. Sometimes an insight needs time to germinate. That requires a patient suffering for fulfillment, somewhat like a gardener planting a late spring crop. Often surprised by new insights, one's Soul is active in creating new roots and foliage as the seed dies to give new life.

Gardening and tending to the cultivation of crops is an example of the ordinary. The image of the fruit tree I discussed earlier only makes sense because I sat with the image and questioned it in the silence of my heart. Images have a voice of their own and need to be heard. It is often difficult for modern people to learn the art of listening to what an image needs to say. So central is the reflection urge within us that Jung maintained it is one of the three psychic energies of the Soul.[89]

It is interesting how these energies pull us beyond their presence so we can participate more intimately with them. The image of a stump with new shoots surrounded by some healthy fertilizer became a portal leading me beyond the image to what the image wished to say. So, what did I need to do to focus on goals for self-care? What did fertilizing my roots mean to me? Jungian analyst Robert Bosnak said it best: the reflection urge leads us beyond the threshold that the image presents and moves us into a world of many possibilities.[90] The following story of David and Robert illustrates the many possibilities that arise when we create space for emerging images that wish to speak to us.

A Caregiver's Nightmare

Daniel's life came to a screeching halt when his phone rang one November morning. His partner had just left for a meeting five minutes before as Daniel was ready to jump into the shower. Something told him to look at his phone. There was a missed message from Robert that said, "Daniel, this is Robert, I'm so sorry, I just crashed the car. I am down the driveway next to the house on the side of the hill, and I called 911, I believe I'm ok." Imagine the different images that raced through Daniel's mind as he dressed, called a friend, and raced to the site as quickly as he could.

In terms of information, Daniel knew only that Robert crashed the car down the hill and that he was ok. It wasn't until he saw the car squeezed into a six-foot-wide space between a garage and a retaining wall that the image of the crash took on a deeper meaning. Paramedics were at the scene when Daniel arrived, and Robert was already in an ambulance. He had quickly exited the car for fear it might explode. The car hit a water faucet on the side of the garage, and water pooled around car. The sight of the car with a broken windshield, crushed fenders, and damaged siding brought Daniel to tears.

The image, like the jaws of Jonah's whale, swallowed him into the darkness of its belly and evoked many possibilities. How did the car get there? What had actually happened? How did Robert get out of the car? Was he seriously hurt? Even more poignantly, how did he survive? Too many questions began cascading into Daniel's consciousness seeking answers. Robert was safe and that was what mattered the most. There was just enough time for a quick hello as the ambulance took off to the hospital. The police and first responders tried to piece together what happened. Daniel would have to wait until he met Robert in the emergency room to discover more answers.

Still in shock after a myriad of tests, Robert tried to recount what happened. When Robert backed up to make a left turn down their driveway, the accelerator stuck, causing the car to race forward. If he continued forward, he drive into a ravine, so he steered the car down the driveway. He tried the brakes, but they did not stop the car. At the end of the driveway across the street there was a storage shed, and behind it, a trailer. Not wanting to harm anyone, Robert steered the car to the right and drove down a steep roadway that led him out of the cul-de-sac. Again, he had no brakes and his speed continued to increase.

Robert was terrified. He clung to the steering wheel for dear life as if riding a bucking bronco at a rodeo, and still trying to gain control, he slid through a wire fence into a field on the right side of the road. Before he knew it, the car hit a ditch on the descending hill and overturned two or three times, sliding into the space between the garage and a retaining wall. Robert said, "I didn't black out, I just held onto the steering wheel with my seat belt fastened, terrified, but still in control." Daniel commented that, in a way, Robert was still in control, Daniel commented, as he did successfully steer the car to safety. In shock, Robert continued, "I knew I had to get out of the car as it was still running."

The impact of the accident echoed through each membrane and muscle of both Daniel and Robert. Using his caregiving instincts, Daniel realized it was time he reached out for help for himself and for Robert. Daniel needed to share with me, a close friend and also a coaching colleague, what happened. As Daniel shared the story, I knew I needed to come over that evening to be with them. My role was simply to be present as best I could and listen.

Impact

The impact of any traumatic shock is felt deep within the body, in muscle memory and in the nervous system. Unlike the instinctual fight or flight response that releases adrenaline and other biochemical reactions, when the body is overwhelmed or blocked by a traumatic experience, the body freezes, trapping all the mobilized survival energy in the body.[91] The family members and spouse of the affected person also vicariously experience the shock, as if the impact happened to them. Daniel, shaking and in tears, kept repeating to me, "I just can't believe he is alive. I'm not ready to lose him." Everyone is impacted by the traumatic event, whether they were there in person or whether they heard the story secondhand. This clearly applies to caregivers, so let's break down this phenomenon to better understand what the caregiver goes through after experiencing a traumatic event, or having the event retold to you, which happened to me.

First, the simple facts of the event can speak volumes and seize one's imagination (recall the different images that raced through Daniel's imagination before he even saw the car accident). Second, each image, like the slides of a PowerPoint, evokes different responses and feelings. They seem to have a life of their own. Some traumatic events may lead one to experience the symptoms of post-traumatic stress, where the chemical triggers of the brain continue to present images of the event as if a film projector was stuck in the brain, unable to shut off, like PTSD.

Trauma expert Diane Poole Heller listed several symptoms that can occur if the threat response, the impact of the accident, is not "completed." These may include anxiety, such as restlessness and excessive energy, feeling disconnected and disoriented, fears of helplessness, hypervigilance, sexual apathy, exhaustion, physical pain, being easily startled, being triggered by similar events, and weight gain.[92]

After the traumatic accident, as Daniel and Robert knew it was a time to debrief, they asked me to become their life coach. With my help, they began to create their new normal, knowing intuitively what was before was shattered and recognizing that the foundation of their relationship, uncannily, had become stronger. Life had not ended, but it certainly changed for both Robert and Daniel. The accident had become a transformative event in their relationship, something that needed to be explored. Something ended that November morning on many levels and something new was beginning. It was in this liminal in-between space, between the ending and a new beginning, where all the answers would be revealed.

Smacked Against a Telephone Pole

Listening to their story challenged me to reflect on my own experiences, an important exercise for every caregiver. Robert and Daniel shared the story of their accident with me, I noticed a faint voice in the background of my consciousness. The voice was seeking an audience about an auto accident I had three years ago. Clearly something about their story was resonating with my own. Both Daniel and Robert were pleased that I could empathize with what they were feeling.

When they asked me how I understood, I told the story of hitting a telephone pole with my car, and the emotional and psychological impact it had on me. I vividly remember my car sliding off an icy road to avoid hitting a deer. Smack! The impact was immediate as I slid into a telephone pole on the side of the curbless road. I felt the pushback from the pole, as it was certainly stronger than a sliding car, and even though I was only going about five miles an hour, the bumper and front right wheel were damaged. Once the car finally stopped, I felt the shock of what had just happened. But how do you really feel the impact and its subsequent shock?

Even now, I can still hear and feel the impact of the crash. My body still reverberates from this experience, something I continue to sort out. How does it feel to drive into a wall—sort of stupid or surprised? Again, smack, like accidentally walking into the glass door of a department store. The impact of hitting the telephone pole was buried deeply in the fibers of my body, yet as I listened to Robert, I realized he had a similar experience. His car hit the side of a garage, mine hit a telephone pole. My feelings had been hidden, but were emerging as I listened and became more empathetic. Maybe Robert also felt stupid, surprised, or confused.

How often do we caregivers feel the traumatic events of others? If these stories remind us of our own traumatic experiences, what do we do? Sometimes we just stuff them down, one after another, until one blindsides us because the accumulation of traumas results in the symptoms of severe compassion fatigue, leading to burnout, secondary stress disorder and even complex PTSD. (Recall when I spoke about the three cultural taboos caregivers face: not to trust, not to share our experiences, and not to share our emotions.) After the event, both Daniel and Robert set aside a block of time each day to explore together what had ended, what they were exploring, and what challenges were emerging in this new beginning. This time for reflection led to more active listening, allowed them to learn from each other, and cultivated a new sense of gratitude for each day. Addressing the experience together also prevented some of the difficult symptoms that could have led to a diagnosis of compassion fatigue, burnout, secondary stress disorder, and complex PTSD.

When You Speak of Soul, You Go Deeper

A relationship with Soul requires us to take time and reflect on the best ways to nourish and sustain ourselves as caregivers. The question for you might be, "Why rush?", but for another, it might be "Why wait?" We need to balance patience with conscious activity, and a relationship with Soul can help us discern whether to act or to sit still.

Reflection is the work of the Soul which gathers and ponders those moments of reverie that connect inner and outer worlds. That is why I chose the pomegranate as a symbol of caregiving, because each caregiver must allow the spark of insight to germinate. Just as the pomegranate reveals its secrets in due season, so too does the Soul refresh with insight and wisdom. Campbell said the work of reflection is the work of a mystic, because Soul penetrates us through the image and symbol. We get lost; time and space seem to disappear. The caregiver enters the land of many possibilities, to a place beyond meaning, to silence, listening to the point of nothingness, where time and eternity meet.[93]

A Seasoned Mentor

Mentors are those in one's profession who are experienced and trusted advisors. There is a generative aspect to a mentor who, because of their learned experience, wishes to guide those who are in the earlier stages of their journey. Mentors can teach younger caregivers the process of reflection, and in a way, that is how they become mentors.

My experience in evaluating different mentorship programs has revealed most programs stress the importance of a mentor to making a commitment to support the growth and development of an interested client by willingly sharing their accumulated knowledge, skills, insights, experience, and wisdom. One such example is Dr. William Potter, a retired obstetrician, who mentored thousands of medical students. Potter shared an experience he had early in his career to emphasize the importance of touch and its sacred ramifications in humanizing medical care. A routine medical examination became the linchpin to understanding his role in becoming sensitive and compassionate to the women he served.

Vulnerability and Ice

Over forty years ago, the young intern William Potter entered a chilly room to complete his first pelvic exam. Nothing was warm about the procedure either—it consisted of a rigid set of protocols, and when Potter entered the room, the patient was already straddled in stirrups, a position which seemed inhumane to Potter and further exacerbated his discomfort. Potter provided explanations to try to ease the apprehension of the patient. What this young student would later remember was the apparent inhumanity, the cold, sterile instruments, and the anonymous cadre of instructors and medical students in attendance. Potter's memory of this image has a life of its own, balancing human vulnerability and the science of medicine. Potter's task, that is, to learn to perform a pelvic examination, was so full of protocols he felt the patient got lost in the shuffle.

I imagine even the most routine of such exams is something most women would rather not have, and I would argue most men have no idea how such an exam borders on a razor-thin line of necessity versus violation, potentially transforming a medical procedure into an intrusive, even traumatic, encounter for the female patient. Needless to say, the memory of this first encounter over forty years ago became the motivation to humanize this procedure in Dr. Potter's practice. He always made sure a female nurse welcomed the patient, reviewed the procedure with her, then prepared her for the examination.

Later in his career, Dr. Potter would also welcome the patient himself and explain each step as he completed the examination. When he teaches medical students, interns, and residents this procedure, Dr. Potter emphasizes the importance of being sensitive to and aware of the patient's feelings. There is an intimacy involved that requires both a professional competency and a caring awareness of the vulnerable nature of the patient. Dr. Potter also shares how he failed to deal with the tension that arose in him during this early experience.

Self-care was not included in Dr. Potter's medical training. He, along with many other physicians I interviewed, described the sense of competition that is rampant among physicians. He explained physicians fear being perceived as incompetent, which may also lead to perfectionistic behaviors, such as refusing to let go of a dying patient and trying everything possible to save them, even if it causes harm to the patient in the process. Physicians are trained to solve the "riddle" of illness, seeking a solution at all costs, even treating when it is futile to do so.[94] In this context, it is even less commonplace to be vulnerable with a trusted friend, teammate, or colleague.

It was often difficult for Dr. Potter to admit his vulnerability regarding a particular case, or the feelings that arose because of it. Stuffing his feelings led to broken relationships and alcoholism, but fortunately, his involvement in Alcoholic Anonymous saved both his life and his career. He is kinder now, not only to his patients but also to himself. He came to realize that the ice that needed to be melted was within himself. Insight was gained from personal reflection on the importance of self-care. The experience was more than an event etched in his memory—it transformed him into the skillful, compassionate doctor he is today. Reflection on his first experience as a medical student over forty years ago, and many subsequent experiences since then, has made Dr. Potter a gifted mentor.

Conclusion

In this chapter, I stressed the importance that we, as caregivers, like the air that we breathe automatically, have the innate skill to reflect on our experiences. We are trained to do it professionally, but more often than not, we spend little time considering how our professional work affects us, and even less time cultivating our Soul's garden. The vignettes in this chapter were examples of the caregiver's experience of reflection. What is the glue, the motivation, the interior strength that sustains caregivers? Can we allow ourselves to acknowledge the good we do and what sustains us in our profession? This question is further developed in our next chapter, which focuses on the spirituality of caregiving.

A Moment of Reflection

At your own pace, give yourself a moment of leisure to reflect on each question below.

1. How would you describe reflection? Can you recognize when you are doing it?

2. As you read through the vignettes in this chapter, did any insights arise?

3. Is reflection a practice that is helpful to you?

4. Do you recognize an ending, a journey, and a new beginning that has happened or is happening to you now?

5. Can you recall an event that transformed you?

_____

_____

_____

_____

_____

_____

_____

_____

_____

_____

_____

_____

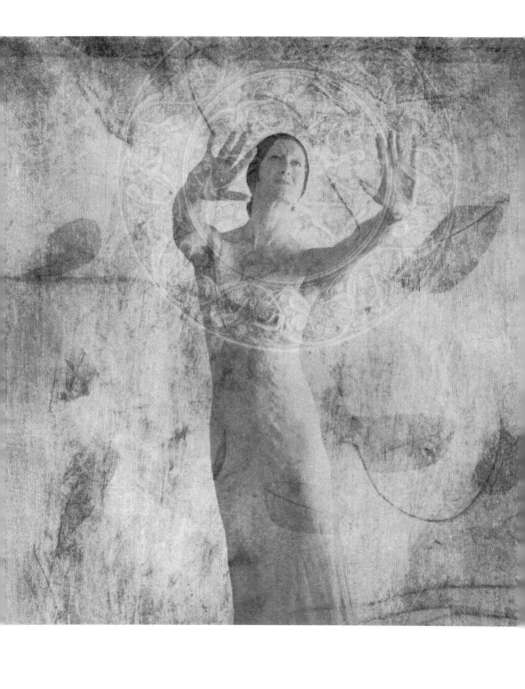

Chapter 8 - Spirituality: The Sinew of our Human Experience

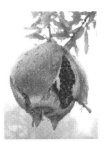

There is nothing objective about spirituality. There may be different shades of gray to its meaning. For some, it is an energizing search for meaning. Others are simply repulsed when spirituality is mentioned, as memories of painful experiences emerge from their past. Still, others are repulsed by the news or experience of the fundamentalist fringes which often seem alive and well within many spiritual and religious traditions. Others simply reject anything spiritual. In general, caregivers are trained to remain neutral, that is, to be hospitable to the spiritual traditions of those they are called to serve. Often, sensitivity to these beliefs helps in building trust, as many studies have shown, a person's spirituality aids in the healing process.[95], [96], [97] In this chapter, I want to introduce the premise that there is a spirituality of caregiving, something that resides deep within the Soul of the caregiver.

Enfleshed Spirituality

The miracle of spirituality is enfleshed in who we are as humankind. Believer and nonbeliever, churched and unchurched, agnostic and atheist, humanist, and theist, we all share a common spirituality: we are human. The sinew, the fibers that hold muscle to bone, is like the balance between flesh and spirit. In this balance of creation, the living principle that permeates our flesh is spiritual, like the air we breathe. The key word is enfleshed, which means the physical is infused with a living energy which we call spirit. Flesh becomes enlivened, which is depicted in the stunning, serene yet dramatic fresco of Michelangelo's interpretation of the Genesis creation story in the Sistine Chapel. Imagine the yearning of Adam, seeking to discover the sacred within himself, reaching out, gazing forward with eyes fixed on the One he is to encounter, extending a hand to be grasped by God. You can feel Adam, eager and receptive, yearning to touch the hand of God. In the synapse between them, the space that is as close as it is distant, life occurs, matter and spirit are joined. Their extended hands become a metaphor for a deeper willingness to share life.

Hands as a Metaphor

Pause for a moment to gaze at your hands. Notice how alive they are. Life pulsates through veins and arteries, feeding cells and exchanging nutrients for waste. Structurally held together by bone and sinew, hands feel warm, sometimes cold, and made able to move by millions of electrically charged neurons. These hands show the fruits of their labor, some with the calluses and bruises of farmers and laborers, others cared for as those of a surgeon, therapist, or nurse, others delicate and fashionable as the principal ballet dancer or violin player, still others with the strength to reach out in friendship with the shake of a hand. Hands whirl flour-dusted pizza dough into the air, create, tailor, and mend our garments, and cook, holding up a wooden spoon to taste a simmering soup.

Hands can both hold one tenderly in an embrace, reassuring, caressing, and making love. God is personified and holds us in the palm of his hands in Hebrew and Christian scriptures. At other times, hands protect and push away, creating personal boundaries; they are ready for self- defense, and they can punish. Hands can be raised in protest, as in a march, or joined together in moments of gratitude, welcoming, and prayer. They clap following experiences and performances of excellence. Hands can be young and not so young, male, female, or nonbinary, some with painted nails and some with broken nails. Others are natural, with different hues of color depicting the cultural diversity of humanity which reminds us not only of the life within them, but also the lives they represent.

Each hand is alive because of the spirit of life that animates them. Spirit, or Soul, is the vital animating essence of a human life, animal life, and vegetal life, as in indigenous spiritual traditions which honor and revere Father Sky and Mother Earth. Spirit is about the non-physical, about the Soul. This broader understanding enables us to imagine spirituality as it relates to this animating energy or force within a person. Spirituality is multifaceted like the hues of a precious gem. Spirituality is about life. It is about living. It is about one's relationship to self, about one's relationship to others and about one's relationship to the Holy Other, the All One. Philosopher Houston Smith described this trinity of relationships and how they are related.[98] For example, if we focus on the transcendent Other, the All One, we will also discover something about ourselves and creation. We may begin our reflection on the beauty of creation, or on our friends or family, and in doing so, we may experience the transcendent Other. Likewise, if we begin to reflect on the miracle of who we are, our real selves, we will discover not only something about ourselves, but also something about creation, others, and the Other.

Spirituality is the living principle, the sinew of our human experience. Sinew, the glue that holds us together, like spirituality. This living principle, the energy that makes us alive, circulates throughout the flesh of our hands. Life lives within us and outside of us, in the world we inhabit, from the heights of the heavens to the depths of the seas to the hills and valleys of the earth. Fruits of the earth, golden waves of planted grains, and dew drenched forests share a common bond with us. So do the creatures of the seas, birds of the air, and creatures of the land breathe the spirit of creation. Each in their own way reminds us that we share with creation the miracle of life. Caregivers sustain life for those they serve, struggling to rescue and protect, and at the same time very much aware that there is a circle of life. Just as there is a beginning when we are born, there is also an ending when we die.

Caregivers Know the Difference

We, as caregivers, know when someone is not alive. When we caress the hand of a grandparent who has just died. We know just as clearly as a surgeon does when a heart stops during surgery and cannot be resuscitated. The life that once circulated and gave color and warmth has left. We know the pain of burying our pet cat or dog in the backyard, or the goldfish that just didn't survive from our own experiences or those of our children or grandchildren. We know the first frost that beautifies and blankets the land with a delicate white will kill flowers or damage crops. Seasons mark these changes and the circle of life continues.

Caregivers face the drama of life and death each day, such as the miracle and joy of delivering a newborn baby or the tragedy and pain of a stillborn child. The satisfaction of saving a life in the emergency room animates the staff and carries them through the sadness when a clinician pronounces someone dead on arrival. The hospice nurse reaches out to a questioning spouse who wonders if life has left and becomes the midwife, tenderly taking the hand of a spouse or friend to comfort when their loved one has died. The parents who, day in and day out, selflessly care for their child with cerebral palsy, celebrating each milestone of achievement, grieve just as deeply as parents who suffer over the premature death of a child, a victim of an opium overdose. What prompts an educator to spend more time with a student she knows will succeed with just a little extra help?

Paramedics and first responders also know the difference between life and death in facing the tragedies of traffic accidents, searching for the victims of floods, wildfires, or hurricanes. They experience the joy of a rescue and the pain of not finding survivors. Their rapid response teams are on alert, ever questioning whether they could have done better. Their debriefing sessions support the recognition that it is difficult to bear human tragedies that leave no one unscathed. What and who sustains these courageous men and women in their service as caregivers? Does their call to service energize them and sustain them through traumatic events? They, like most caregivers, would agree that something greater than themselves sustains them, yet few would recognize or call what they do a spiritual practice. But what if we entertain the possibility that this energizing and animating spirit of one's call to service could also be called spirituality?

Is the work of caregiving just a job or is it a calling, and as such, can we reimagine caregiving as a spiritual practice? We are not going to a church, synagogue, mosque, monastery, or an ashram, nor are we going to our prayer circle or gathering in the wilderness. We don't need our bible, holy scriptures, prayer beads, prayer shawl, or chants. Our journey is an interior one, where spirit and flesh meet It is at this juncture, where spirit and flesh meet, that insight is gained. Imagine this life-giving force circulating throughout your body sustaining you as a caregiver.

Holding What Cannot Be Held

How does one hold what seems to be unbearable for both caregivers and those they serve? Consider the experience of Chaplain Richards, a seasoned member of the interdisciplinary team at a trauma one medical center who, like the director of a one-act tragedy, was called to the emergency room. Mr. Brown was on his way to the hospital because he had suffered a massive cardiac arrest at home. He was an elder at the First Baptist Church in his community, and members of his family sang in the choir. He was the glue that held his large African-American family together. He and his family were celebrating the birthday of one of their grandchildren, laughing and playing games, when Mr. Brown suddenly fell to the floor. One of his daughters who was an RN rushed to his side and began cardiopulmonary resuscitation (CPR), while his son called 911. His wife, trying to keep her composure, escorted the children to another room. Within minutes, the paramedics took over, continuing CPR, taking vital signs, communicating with the ER physician, starting an IV and administering cardiac medications. The call to service was immediate for Chaplain Richards, the ER physician, and the paramedics. Still doing CPR on arrival, the emergency room staff continued to no avail, and he was pronounced dead shortly after his arrival.

Most of the family of Mr. Brown followed the ambulance to the emergency room, while a daughter remained at home with the children. They were greeted by Chaplain Richards, who led them to the ER family room. He had already been informed of the situation by the ER staff. Their panic and apprehension were increased as they wondered why a chaplain would greet them. Years of training prepared Chaplain Richards to face such situations. Calmly, he reassured the family that this was the protocol of the hospital in emergency situations, and the doctor had asked him to help get the family settled until he could come and speak with them. He told them the situation was serious and that the doctor will be in shortly. "Is he going to live?" shouted one of his daughters. A prediction only the doctor could confirm, a decision Chaplin Richards was gently preparing the family to hear. "It is very grave," he replied. Tearfully, she mentioned that on the way to the hospital, her mother called their pastor and he too, was on his way.

Clearly, the family was in shock, tearful and anxious, as they realized the patriarch and elder of their family, a spouse, a father, and grandfather, may die. How does one hold what no one wants to acknowledge? Would their spirituality support them and be a resource to them? Within this tension of holding the tragedy and the suffering and woundedness, is there a possibility of discovering healing and transformation, something that evokes at least symbolic death and new awareness.[99] One's response to trauma or woundedness gradually leads to this letting go, a sort of dying and rising or what we discussed earlier by William Bridges: an ending, uncertainty, and a new beginning. This was the process the Brown family would face.

Facing the end of a loved one's life may, in time, become a life-giving and transformative experience. Bearing what appears to be unbearable, feeling the seemingly endless pain, walking into the depths our netherworld and allowing the darkness to surround us are all steppingstones in the process of descent. Every individual can bear the pain and find their way through the labyrinth of the Soul that seeks transformation. This was the certitude Chaplain Richards experienced as he witnessed the Brown family entering this mystery—not only was a husband and father dying, but something within each family member was being transformed.

Chaplain Richards reassured the family he would keep them informed as he went to check with the doctor, who had already pronounced Mr. Brown dead. The doctor asked if he should now come and speak with the family. Chaplain Richards suggested he wait until Mr. Brown's pastor arrived, due to the family's need for support and their strong spiritual ties with their Church. Just then, the pastor arrived and was met by Chaplin Richards, who briefed him on the doctor's findings and escorted him to the family conference room.

As soon as Pastor Williams entered the room, there was an outburst of emotion. He shared with the family how grave he believed the situation was and led them in prayer for strength. It was then the doctor arrived and compassionately told the family that Mr. Brown had essentially died at home due to a traumatic cardiac arrest. He expressed his condolences and left the room. In the meantime, the nurses were preparing Mr. Brown to be seen by his family. Pastor Williams embraced Mrs. Brown, whose glistening tears streamed through the aged wrinkles of her mahogany complexion. Each of the children surrounded their mother in a circle of compassion and grief. Ernie, the oldest of the five children, recognized his new role: to support his mother and his other siblings. Then, he asked what was next.

Chaplain Richards asked if anyone in the family would like to see Mr. Brown and he would escort them, a few at a time, into the ER proper. Afterwards, Mr. Brown would be taken to the hospital morgue until the funeral director was chosen. Papers needed to be signed, giving permission for the hospital to release the remains to the funeral director who would be in touch with the family. Each person involved relied on and was supported by a different understanding of spirituality that sustained them during this traumatic event. The paramedics, the doctor, the chaplain, the ER staff, the pastor, and the family each held on, sometimes blindly, sometimes unnerved, and sometimes with a steel and steadfast faith, because of their spiritual roots and their spirituality. So, what is spirituality?

The Many Facets of Spirituality

While spirituality is often equated with a formalized religious practice, the Sacred and Divine, the supernatural, the afterlife, and religious traditions and practices, its essence lies at the center of being human. Spirituality is as natural as breathing. (Many spiritual traditions even incorporate breathing practices in their rituals.)

Spirituality may also find its expression in nature, humanism, psychology, philosophy, the arts, and religious practice. Breathing in and breathing out is a conscious and unconscious rhythm of uniting the elements of the earth with the elements of the sky, the physical and spiritual, at the center of one's being. Breathing in and breathing out is humankind's universal experience of common ground, of awareness of being one with the All One and one with all beings and creation.

As there is movement in the exercise of breathing, so too is spirituality an animating force of change and movement within a person.[100] As such, our call to action as caregivers is often guided by our spiritual values, or what I like to call a spirituality of caregiving. Breathing in and breathing out restores wellness and hope, of catching our breath, accepting the gift of life-giving air within the deepest caverns of our Soul. Spirit enters and is united with our personal spirit, which energizes us. Breathing out, exhaling, is a metaphor of "spiriting" one to serve those in need. A healer of body, mind, and spirit, breath unites each caregiver with the human drama of illness, wellness, suffering, and the comfort in being at ease with both the miracles and limitations of caregiving.

From a Depth-Psychological Perspective

Understanding spirituality as a natural urge within a person's psyche was developed by Austrian founder of psychoanalysis, Sigmund Freud, and the Swiss founder of analytical psychology, C. G. Jung. These natural urges are not tangible, not in the sky, not in the supernatural, but in the natural essence of being human. As previously mentioned, to be human is to be enfleshed, to be united in matter and spirit. For Westerners raised in a culture that separates the logos and mythos of the human experience from each other, this is a difficult concept to understand. This is not to say they are literally united, but rather, it simply means that within the human experience, in the physical boundaries that contain who I am, I can and do experience transcendence. This is why I marveled at Campbell's response to the student who asked the question, "Where is heaven?"[101]

Let's explore Campbell's response again, but substitute the word heaven for "the sacred," "the Holy Other," or "spirituality." Campbell said: "Is it above? Then the birds will be there before you. Is it below? Then the fish will be there before you. The Kingdom of God is within you. Who and what is in Heaven? God is in Heaven. Where is God? Within you!"[102] Eastern spiritualities start with this premise of humanity and spiritual experience. We in the West go through the back door to arrive at the same conclusion. In the Christian Tradition, how often can we recall Jesus saying, "The kingdom of God is within you"?

Suspended between inner and outer, earth and sky, above and below, resides the meeting place where Sacred and Divine, humankind, and the mysteries of the universe become one. "Thou art That!" articulates the message as well as it can, epitomizing the unity with the Divine, which resides not only within the individual but is identical with a universal, absolute consciousness of the sacred. This meeting point or threshold is the language of metaphor and is where mystics roam and see reality differently. Metaphor, like the discipline of prayer, becomes the portal by which the seeker journeys beyond the historical fact to an experience that transcends human experience. Jungian analyst Lionel Corbett articulated this experience: "This non-dual notion of the Self expresses in psychological language the mystical understanding that, in [Meister] Eckhart's words, 'my me is God,' or as the Upanishads of the Hindu myths put it, 'thou art that.'"[103]

The experience is not outside of ourselves but within. For example, if I was raised in a Western culture derived from the Greek and Roman influences, I would probably consider the sacred outside of myself. There is me and there is the sacred other, distinctly separate from me.

Freud was averse to using the term "spiritual," as he equated it with religion. Again, wanting to stress the normalness of humanity that he found in these spiritual urges, he used the German word *seele*. Translated, it means an embodied Soul which contains within it all the natural instincts needed for self-actualization, a process of clarifying who we are destined to be. [104] Could we argue that his understanding of the interior process is spiritual, as is our own natural spirituality, just as we understand the naturalness of flesh and spirit in our hands?

Jung also realized this natural urge toward self-actualization, as well as the psychic energies that drive it, are intrinsic to being human. He called this process "individuation," the process of a person discovering and becoming their true self, which involves both the individual and the collective unconscious. Unlike Freud, Jung suggested that within this natural urge, there is also a transcendent quality which leads one to reflect beyond oneself. This led Jung to define spirituality as the "careful and scrupulous observation of the numinosum."[105] Gaining insight from our reflections is something we do every day. Amid these reflections one may experience the sacred. For example, as we witness the sun rising over the hills and valleys, or the sun setting into the Pacific Ocean, we may sense God or the Holy Other is the creator of this panorama of color, or we may understand this phenomenal moment as sacred in and of itself. In doing so, almost without any effort, we experience what Jung called the numinosum, which simply means the presence of a divinity, something spiritual, something awe-inspiring. Specifically, Jung understood numinosity in the context of archetypes, which are universal patterns with corresponding instinctual behaviors and attitudes. Caregiving is an example of a pattern of behavior that influences the work we do with a certain attitude, or as I have suggested, a certain calling as a nurse, a first responder, an educator, physician, homecare maker, parent, spouse or firefighter.

A Caregiver's Spirituality

Caregivers contain the resources necessary for interior reflection, and they are influenced by values that often effect how they view their calling. Recall how those in the healing professions live out archetypes such as the Wounded Healer, the Caregiver, or the Hero. Each profession has a unique culture and archetypal pattern that reminds them they belong to something bigger than their individual self. What does it mean to be a police officer or a detective belonging to a fraternal order of police committed to living out the pledge of the "Blue Line" that separates legal and illegal activities? The collective consciousness of the group encompasses values and beliefs that support and encourage its members in their search for meaning.

Another definition of spirituality caregivers may experience is one suggested by Robert Grant. According to Grant, spirituality "is grounded in the ability to foster relationship, to be connected, and to be whole. Wholeness requires embracing dimensions of inner and outer reality that life outside has been 'taken for granted.'"[106] The very act of caregiving is relational, a meeting between the caregiver and the one being served, as well as our relationship to the event and how it affects us. There is always the tension of applying our professional and technical skills to a situation, our relationship with who we are serving, our team members, and our relationship with ourselves.

Discovering and understanding the different movements of his Soul, let alone following through on them, was new for Duston, nicknamed Dusty. As a vice-president of human resources (HR), Dusty discovered he took relationships for granted and often dismissed his relationship with himself, his family, and his spiritual life, which he had inherited as the son of a Congregational minister.

The Son of a Preacher Man

As early as Dusty can remember, he was always a caregiver. Inspired by his father, who was pastor of a progressive nondenominational Congregational church. Dusty often tagged along with his parents, brother, and sister at each church function, and as he grew older, he volunteered to help with various outreach programs in the community. He felt a particular sensitivity and compassion for the underserved. He enjoyed serving meals in the church soup kitchen, as well as belonging to the youth group who went on missions to poorer areas of the country. It would be years before Dusty realized this sensitivity was borne out of his own unconscious need to care for himself, something he did not learn at home. There is a negative side to caregiving: sometimes the obsessive need to help others is an unconscious attempt to muffle the cry of a caregiver's Soul pain.

What Dusty couldn't reconcile or understand was his parent's use of recreational drugs. It just didn't make sense to him, as they were well-respected leaders in the community, known for their empathy and pastoral concern. This quandary would eventually lead him to leave the Church. What was missing in his parent's lives? And, more importantly, what was missing in Dusty's life? His father, the pastor, would smoke marijuana before each service. He later learned his grandfather died of cirrhosis of the liver due to alcoholism, and it would be years later, when confronted with his own addiction, that Dusty identified the intergenerational pattern of addictive behaviors within his family of origin. He learned addictive behaviors mask one's real need to form relationships. Dusty learned caregiving, though enriching, also has a negative side. The negative aspects of caregiving are observed in individuals who, consciously or unconsciously, psychologically identify with the archetypal Martyr or Victim; they are unable to say no, and enable the self-destructive behaviors of others. Additionally, caregivers often suffer from codependency, perfectionism, and feel an ever-present sense of guilt due to a lack of accomplishment, even if they have personally or professionally accomplished a great deal.

A Professional Juggler

As vice president of HR for a large telecommunications company, Dusty found himself assuming a variety of roles with the many associates who came to his office. One day, he found himself consoling an associate whose husband was killed in an car accident. Another day, he listened to a disgruntled director having a bad hair day. Still another, he worked with his team organizing the annual employee picnic. He enjoyed this aspect of his job as an informal social worker, pastoral counselor, and financial advisor, always having one or two balls in the air, as he prided himself on being a juggler. Long hours, however, began to take a toll on him, as well as the unending organizational demands of his job. He got the nickname "Dusty" early on because of his golden-brown hair, but in a way, he enjoyed being the dust mop of the organization, cleaning up other people's issues.

To keep himself going, Dusty would have two or three martinis at the end of each day. Little did he know he had inherited the addictive behaviors of his parents. In a college course, Dusty had to draw a genogram, which is like a family tree, except that it focuses on the emotional, social, spiritual, and psychological dynamics in a family. What he learned (but didn't take to heart) was that he could trace addictive behaviors not only in his parents, but to five preceding generations. There was also a pattern of the men in the family dying early, and the resultant anger and resentment of the wives forced to live on alone. He also learned there was a strong reliance on faith—not only was his father a pastor, but also his father's father. The question then arose for Dusty: What was missing in each of their lives, and now even in his own? Why didn't their spiritual practice support them in this process? As an adult, he left formalized religious practice to seek answers to these questions.

Blessings and Pitfalls

Although the caregiver has many strengths, the caregiver can also fall victim to what Pearson referred to as "pitfalls."[107] Dusty was well known in the company for his compassion and being one whose door was always open. As best he could, he tried to model the leadership qualities of "servant leadership."[108] His duties as an HR executive made him an advocate both for the associates who sought his help and at the executive table where he helped promote policies for them. What Dusty didn't recognize were the pitfalls he would stumble into which developed from his generous heart. He often felt overwhelmed, going in so many directions, unable to say no to demands from the executive leadership office and the demands from the associates. He often felt like a martyr for the cause, sword in hand, ready for the battle cry.

Codependency and enabling others are behaviors inherent in addictive personalities, which he later recognized. It was as ludicrous as someone hosting a cocktail party to celebrate their sobriety. He learned early that he should not upset the applecart at home. If one member of a household takes the risk of self-improvement and growth, the family system is affected, and the resistance of the other family members builds, often to sabotage the one seeking recovery. This was one of the reasons, while not fully conscious, that Dusty withdrew from his church and family. He however, continued to carry his intergenerational wounds or baggage.

If one takes on too much, maybe trying to fill a personal interior void, then one has little time for self-care. If one never feels good enough, then it is possible not to set healthy boundaries. Resentment and guilt can build up, creating a craving for a good old fashioned "pity party." However, this does not undermine the core values and qualities of the caregiver such as nurturance, compassion, dedication, generosity, service, and personal sacrifice for the good of others. The qualities of being supportive, kind, helpful, altruistic, caring, and concerned with the well-being of others are still core competencies and skills.[109] Dusty recognized he could identify with many of these caregiver core values and strengths. He also recognized the pitfall of being a martyr and lacking in self-care. If only he cared enough, if only he had done more; "If only" became his mantra until one day he ran out of gas. He became a caretaker instead of a caregiver, and the emptiness he experienced was filled with alcohol.

A Balm in Gilead

In his search for answers, Dusty realized he was an alcoholic, which became his "Balm in Gilead," the refrain of an African American spiritual he remembered when he was in the youth group at this father's church. However, he realized he was substituting alcohol for a deeper opportunity for self-awareness and relationship building. Intuitively, Dusty was searching for meaning and healing which he did not find being the son of a preacher-man. The route he took, the balm he sought, the tonic he thought would refresh him, did not heal, as living on the surface of things did not address his real Soul pain, which was being drowned with alcohol. He yearned for what the spiritual song promised: "There is a Balm in Gilead that makes the wounded whole. There is a Balm in Gilead that heals the sin-sick Soul."[110]

It is often said that though a person may leave a particular spiritual practice, such as going to church, mosque, meeting room, or synagogue, the person's spirituality continues to reside deep within their consciousness, always ready for deeper and richer growth. This realization hit Dusty's consciousness like a thunderbolt one day at work. It had become clear that he needed to write his resignation letter and resign. Years of caregiving had taken their toll, with little or no time for self-care. He was suffering from compassion fatigue leading to burnout (which will be explored further in Chapter Ten). Patricia Smith argued compassion fatigue occurs when we neglect the physical, psychological, interpersonal, and spiritual needs that help us cope with the stress of caregiving.[111] Dusty often said to himself, "There is so much to be done!" which led him to disregard his own need for self-care. However, Dusty felt a flicker of hope, and it was on the strength of this experience that he went to see Dan White, a pastoral counselor specializing in addiction, whom he had previously met at an HR conference. He was impressed with Dan's sincerity and his informal invitation to call him if he ever needed help.

After a month of visiting Dan three times a week, Dusty asked him, "How long will it take to get back on my feet?" There was a pause, and then Dan gently responded, "Dusty, it's not a matter of 'Zap! Bam! Alakazam!' or drinking another tonic. It's about facing a new normal, a new lifestyle, a new recognition that you are now on a journey of healing which will continue for the rest of your life." Dusty nodded in agreement, feeling somewhat relieved, as Dan verified what Dusty was intuitively feeling: he could rely on his spiritual strength, which had become an integral part of Dusty's DNA. At the root of many addictive behaviors is fear of building relationships, and Dusty now discovered that, in trusting Dan, he was also discovering and recovering the relationship he so desired with himself.

Relationships and Spirituality

Spirituality encompasses an awareness of relationship with all creation, as well as an appreciation of presence and purpose that includes a sense of meaning. Thomas Berry, a scholar of world religions, argued a divine presence dwells intimately in the world of creation, which carries a refinement of emotion and sensitivity inspired by the delicacy, fragrance, indescribable beauty, and rhythmic movement of the world.[112] Art, poetry, music, literature, dance, theater, and life's experiences may lead us to reflect, to contemplate, and embrace a mystical sensibility. Mysticism is not reserved for saints, shamans, and sages alone, nor is mysticism outside the realm of the ordinary.

The question then becomes: As a caregiver, am I aware that I participate in many different and unique relationships with my clients, myself, and the sacred? The Hindu revelation that you are it, or "Thou Art That," led Campbell to the awareness that the gods are a projection of one's own inner fire: "Follow the footsteps to your center and know that from within you, gods are born. The deities are symbolic personifications of the energy that you are yourself. Within you is where the gods dwell."[113] The reverential Sanskrit salutation "Namaste," which is found in many Hindu and Asian traditions, articulates this profound truth: the divine within me bows to the divine within you.[114]

"Thou Art That" articulates that the Divine, and the hero's quest the individual yearns for, resides not only within the individual but is also identical to a universal, sacred consciousness. This meeting point or threshold can only be described in the language of metaphor, and within this realm, we can see reality with the eyes of the mystic. Through his travels, research, and reflections, Campbell discovered a universal unity shared among the myths of the world. He was able to see beyond all their distinctive facts and cultural boundaries to the vitalizing energy that each symbol or myth signifies.[115] This is the latent energy we possess as caregivers.

Spirituality and Transcendence

Transcendence is an experience that takes us outside of ourselves as the active participants in the everyday life. The art of contemplation may open us up to mystery and a process of reflection which instantly moves us out of an "either/or" box. Sages, tricksters, mystics, priests, rabbis, Imams, and shamans experience the sacred and mirror this experience from an insider's view. Ordinary reflection creates the conditions that make contemplative reflection possible. Then, the process of exploration and reflection becomes a transformative act, allowing one to experience the sacred. An experience of the sacred is borne out of our human experience—in a sense, it is our birthright as human beings. The task for caregivers is to give themselves permission to allow these insights to develop, percolate, and manifest. Reflection is the beginning of self-care which is the antidote to compassion fatigue.

17th century Italian sculptor Gian Lorenzo Bernini's sculpture of the "Rapture of St. Theresa" in Santa Maria Victoria Church in Rome invites the viewer to enter the artist's realization that solid marble can reflect and evoke human experience. One wonders what inspired Bernini to enliven marble with what he experienced within himself. What was stirring in his Soul, as he got lost in that moment in time, when eternity opened up before him? A moment outside the constraints of time and space captivated Bernini and fueled his struggle to articulate one raptured in love. This work of art acts as a potential portal to the experience of transcendence for us, the viewers, but as dramatic as this work of art is, are there not stories that need to be carved from within us? Don't we contain artful life experiences, insights, and wisdom that, when shared, can support and sustain us as caregivers?

Reflection allows caregivers to see through the symbols and images of our experiences. For a moment, we see beyond the curtain of uncertainties that separates us from the sacred. One who was once outside is now inside this sacred sanctuary as outer and inner merge. What appeared to be distant and unclear melts within the radiance of the present moment. Barriers that once separated mortals from the Sacred and Divine are shattered in the numinosity of the experience. Mystics and spiritual leaders remind us that we too share in this human experience of reflection which allows us to see and understand, in the silence of our being, the place where time and space disappear.

The field of comparative religion is born out of the tension of different perspectives. Religion becomes another view or lens to use in understanding the transcendent experience of a people and a culture. An observation about a particular faith tradition by an anthropologist, psychologist, mythologist, or comparative religionist is an outsider's view, in that they do not practice or participate in the mythos of that faith tradition. Sensitivity to an insider view does add a unique and powerful view. Paden wrote, "much more specific to religion than cognitive representation is the participatory character of meanings and symbols."[116] These symbols also transform perception, and in doing so, engage the participant. Such was the experience of Maria, who, despite relying on her faith, felt fearful and anxious prior to her open-heart surgery. As she was prepared for surgery, she asked the nurse if she could see the chaplain. Conscious of the importance of a patient's well-being and how this contributes to the overall successful outcome of the surgery, the nurse reassured Maria and called the chaplain. Maria was about to discover how much she was a participant in her own recovery.

Caught in the Cauldron of Anxiety and Fear

Sinking in a cauldron of anxiety and fear, Maria called upon the resources of her faith and prayers to assist her, but to no avail. She became even more anxious and asked the nurse to call the chaplain for support. Maria, a seventy-year-old woman of the Roman Catholic faith, specifically asked for a priest. After the normal introductions, Maria greeted the chaplain with the words: "I am praying to God that I will not be anxious about the surgery, yet I am still anxious." Struggling to use her faith and interior resources to cope with her anxiety, she found herself falling into a despair so powerful that she even considered postponing her surgery.

While exploring Maria's particular anxieties about the surgery, such as pain management, what the doctor and nurses had previously told her, her length of stay, possible complications, and even her fear of dying, the chaplain asked almost matter-of-factly: "Did you ever consider just telling God you were anxious?" Maria looked at the chaplain with amazement: "I could actually tell God what I'm feeling?" This was a new insight for her. A wave of calm washed over Maria, as the suggestion that a merciful and compassionate God could possibly understand her feelings, shattered her image of a distant God.

Allowing this new image of God to speak on its own terms became a process of transformation and healing for Maria. The image of a God for whom she had to struggle to get things right transformed into an image of a faithful, loving, compassionate, and merciful God. In the Song of Songs in the Hebrew Scriptures, God is portrayed as a Divine Lover. Within the Christian tradition, images of a God "who so loved the world" emerge in the Gospel of

John. Similarly, within the Sufi tradition of Islam, God is imaged as the Beloved.

Anxiety about open-heart surgery is certainly normal and to be expected, yet Maria's own demons tied her up in knots. Amid these personal demons, she knew she could rely on the wisdom that emerged in her relationship with the chaplain. A spiritual guide had appeared in the person of the chaplain and a restoration of her faith led her to put her anxieties in perspective. The sacrament of the sick was administered, and the chaplain accompanied her to the doors of the surgery suite. When she woke up in intensive care after surgery, the chaplain was there doing his rounds. As he approached and took her hand, she smiled, squeezed his hand, and simply said, "Thank you."

The lesson Maria learned during her hospital stay was that the supernatural is not outside of human experience. Understanding the transcendent as a supernatural phenomenon is only possible if understood from this human perspective. Religion and religious practices then become an expression of one's natural, innate spirituality. Jung believed that since God is an archetype, He already has a place in the deepest center of our psyche which is preexistent to consciousness: "We neither make Him more remote nor eliminate Him but bring Him closer to the possibility of being experienced."[117]

It is often during and after the experience of a traumatic event that one can discover how and when the sacred can be experienced. This is the challenge for caregivers and for those we are called to serve.

Trauma as Soul Building

When a caregiver experiences a traumatic event, the impact of the event is seared within their Soul and has conscious and unconscious effects. Some experiences are so serious they leave us almost paralyzed with fear; specifically, fear that the traumatic event might continually recur. Some experiences are, in relative terms, milder; caregivers can push these experiences aside and get on to the next task. Trauma may also reactivate old patterns which were hidden: traumas experienced as a child or later in life might suddenly appear, almost to haunting us, like a ghostly voice seeking to be heard. Other traumas may suddenly "awaken" in the caregiver, and the subsequent emotional outburst helps the caregiver realize the depth of suffering from an accumulation of traumatic events (perhaps due to an accumulation of "milder" traumatic events, as mentioned above). At this point, the Soul has had enough—it is in pain and its voice will be heard. Fortunately, each aching fiber of Soul pain can guide us on our journey to find appropriate support.

Psychologist Robert Grant defined trauma as "an overwhelming life event(s) that renders most people powerless and/or living in fear of their life. The major challenge of trauma is to integrate its impact into personal and collective frames of meaning."[118] According to Grant, the task or challenge is to find meaning in our afflictions. Jung believed this is one of the functions of the psyche. In allowing the experience of pain to be felt, one may experience wisdom hidden within, maintaining that "Tears, sorrow, and disappointment are bitter, but wisdom is the comforter in all psychic suffering.[119] As Hillman suggested, "Afflictions point to gods; gods reach us through afflictions."[120]

Jungian analyst Greg Mogenson observed: "Compared to the finite nature of the traumatized Soul, the traumatic event seems infinite, all-powerful, and wholly other."[121] In reaction to traumatic events, we often close ourselves off from experiencing the full range of pain engendered by the experience, but only when the trauma is fully felt through a kind of death and resurrection experience can we enter the process of Soul-making, like the mollusk encasing an irritant in layers of protective fluid that gradually transform it into a luminous pearl.[122] What begins as a painful, seemingly destructive invasion becomes a shining, beautiful creation. Wisdom is gained though and not despite our suffering.

The Spirituality of Caregiving

Our discussion of spirituality has led us to discover that the goals, aspirations, commitment, passion, values, and dedication we share as caregivers are steeped in a spirituality of caregiving. Just as the air we breathe is a metaphor for welcoming the sacred or divine host into the core of our being through the gentle act of inhalation, the act of exhalation is a metaphor for our subsequent movement into the world to be of service to others. The ancient exhortation and dismissal from the Catholic Mass, "Ite missa est" says it best, as you have experienced healing transformation during this sacred ritual, so go forth and serve others. Breathing in and out is a simple example of the interchange between flesh and spirit, between a sacred encounter and the commission to serve those in need. We are fed emotionally and spiritually when we do the work of caregiving.

The question I asked in an earlier chapter, which I always ask at the beginning of any lecture or workshop, is: "Are you a better person because of your work as a caregiver?" Most attendees nod their heads in agreement and then move onto the next call or the next patient. The real question is: "As caregivers, are we open to the transformative possibilities that occur because of the work we do?" When we listen to the movements of our Soul, we recognize our work is interior as much as it is exterior. Just as we are fed by this reflective process and experience a sense of spirituality at it foundational roots, so too, do we have the privilege to drink from the fountain of caregiving. This feeding, or tending to our Soul's garden, nourishes us in the careers that make us whole. The work we do is a spiritual practice.

Dr. Christina Puchalski, the founder and director of George Washington Institute of Spirituality and Health (GWISH), has committed her entire career to studying, researching, and advocating for the importance of spirituality in healthcare. GWISH stresses the importance of recognizing the spiritual dimension of both health and suffering. Puchalski argued spirituality is the dimension of a person that seeks to find meaning in their life; spirituality is also the quality that supports connection to and relationship with the sacred, as well as with one another. If this is so, how does the work we do build a connection to and a relationship with the ones we serve? The previously discussed notion of caregivers as wounded healers allows us to reimagine the act of caregiving as being directly related to how we integrate spirituality in the work we do.

Puchalski suggested that as physicians and healthcare workers become more aware of the importance of the spiritual needs of the sick and suffering, their work will become more compassionate and caring. The interaction between physicians, nurses, chaplains, social workers, therapists, auxiliary support personnel and those who are ill demands self-sacrifice and compassion. Such interactions become a spiritual practice. Herein lies the underlying thesis of this work: Caregivers are trained to recognize the spiritual needs of those they serve, but they also discover, participate in, and are animated by their spirituality of caregiving.

Spirituality is an important resource when one experiences different traumatic events in life. The integration of spirituality, caregiving, and health is an ancient practice which continues to motivate healthcare workers, academics, first responders, home healthcare assistants, and family educators.

In a task force called Spirituality, Culture and End of Life Care, Puchalski and her colleagues made recommendations that were included in "Report III, Contemporary Issues in Medicine: Communication in Medicine of the Medical School Objective Project (MSOP)." The report emphasized the importance and necessity of the physician developing communication skills in supporting and facilitating a conversation about a patient's spirituality.[123] The report also recognized that spirituality is found in all cultures and contributes to health in many persons.

Spirituality is expressed in an individual's search for ultimate meaning through participation in religion and/or belief in God, family, naturalism, rationalism, humanism, and the arts. It is important to note that each of these factors can influence how patients and healthcare professionals perceive health and illness, as well as how they interact with one another.[124] But the question remains: "How do we, as caregivers, discover a spirituality that is truly our own?" We don't have to look outside ourselves, to the heavens or the depths below. What we so desire, a spirituality that supports and sustains us, is within us. The key that unlocks this mystery is within our hands. It is a matter of allowing the stirrings of our Soul to be heard. And it is about developing a spiritual practice.

In our next chapter, "Practice, Practice, Practice" I explore what a spiritual practice is and how caregiving is such a practice. For a moment, consider how we must create space and be hospitable enough to welcome the client or the patient. These are spiritual actions. The ordinary becomes spiritual as we discover, through our journey, the interior strengths and values that give birth to meaning, insight, and transformation.

A Moment of Reflection

If you feel you are standing on your head, and that your worldview about spirituality is in transition, or that you are ready to scream, wonderful! You are at a good place. Now, it is time to catch your breath and allow what is stirring have a voice.

When you are ready, here are some questions to ponder. Take your time—this is NOT a test. It is about you and what you have learned about listening to the stirrings of your Soul.

1. You belong to a noble profession. How has reading through this chapter assisted you in more appreciating the work you do?

2. Were you able to gain insight from the different stories presented in this chapter? Can you identify with any of the characters?

3. How has the discussion about trauma and traumatic events helped you to realize you are not alone in experiencing these events as a caregiver?

4. How do you understand the relationship between spirituality and caregiving?

_____

_____

_____

_____

_____

_____

_____

_____

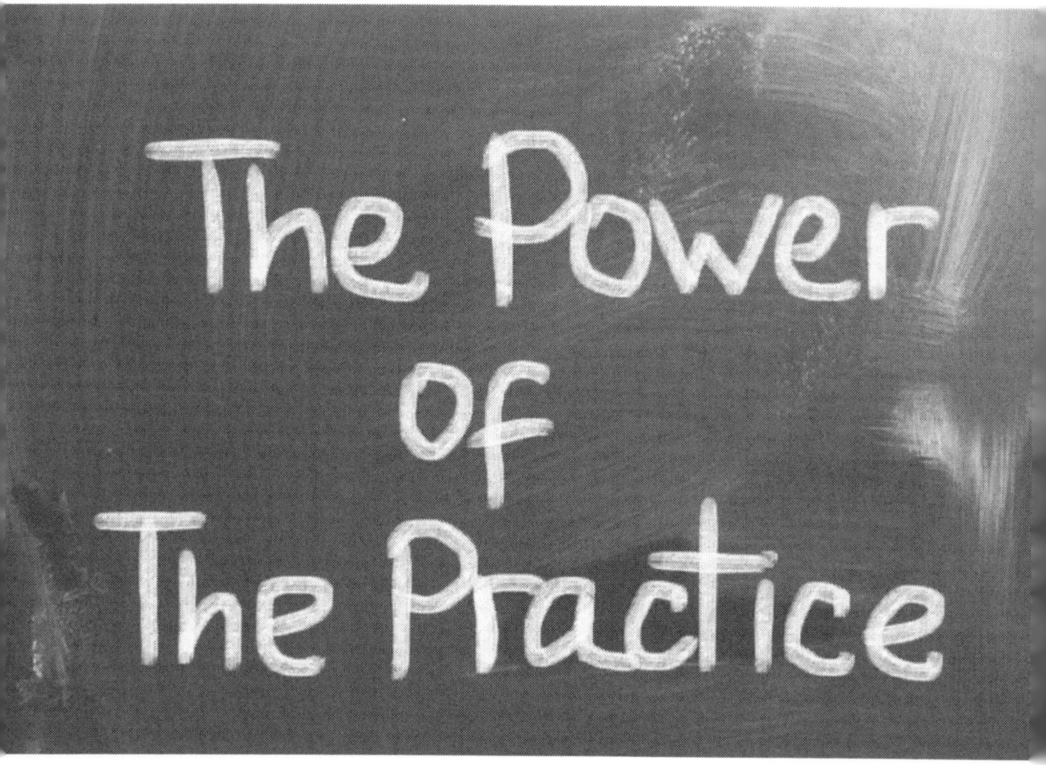
The Power
of
The Practice

Chapter 9 – Practice! Practice! Practice!

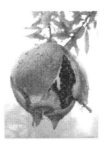

It's time to practice. How often has this word conjured up both excitement and resistance within us? Practice is embedded in our genes, seeking to bring what lies dormant within us to fruition. Conscious and unconscious stirrings both from interior or exterior promptings motivate us to excel, to move forward and to succeed. From our earliest years, from the exuberance of taking our first stumbling steps to the joys of learning the alphabet, to experiencing both the constraints and the rewards of parental guidance.

Practice helps to make us feel more confident in what we are doing. How many arguments did we have or continually have with parents, coaches, instructors, and professors about the importance of practice, especially when we were the least motivated? The concert pianist didn't just appear on the stage, dropping down from the heavens to play on celestial keys, but spent many hours of practice to sharpen her skills. Likewise, those who are fortunate enough to make the Olympic teams do so because of hours and hours of tedious, committed practice. A spark within these aspirants guides them to become Olympic champions.

We of lesser fame may need more time to learn musical scales, even when at times we wonder why we chose to play flute in the first place. What about all those extra push-ups we did when we tried out for sports teams? (Or was it just to tune up and tighten our glutes?) How many extra sprints did we have to run around the varsity track, sometimes to the point of exhaustion, to achieve our goals? For us swimming enthusiasts, how many times did we almost drown before we felt proficient in the freestyle or the breaststroke? What about the hours of voice lessons and rehearsals we endured in the school and college chorus before we could perform? A friend of mine, commenting on how much she devoted to practice, recalled playing the score of Swan Lake on her flute almost a thousand times before her debut, which resulted in a standing ovation after her performance.

Practice is what we caregivers do, and it is part of the learning curve each of us masters to be proficient in our chosen profession. Do you remember how nervous you felt as a student nurse or medical student the first time you gave an injection? Do you remember how difficult it was to scale barricades or carry fire hoses during your first days of training to be a firefighter or the first time you had to pull out your gun in an arrest? How did you feel on your first run as a paramedic? Were you comfortable in being called a "rookie" the first time on the job? How did you feel as a student teacher facing thirty-five fifth graders? How many pieces of paper are crumbled and thrown on the floor in the process of writing an essay or an article? What about the hours of internship training most caregivers must complete for licensure or certification?

Training and internships help us to deepen our skills, to gain insight, and become more efficient through practice. Practice also helps us learn from our mistakes as we gain wisdom through trial and error. When an activity is diligently repeated, skills are honed and developed. Such was the experience of Dale, an art therapist who was a member of an interdisciplinary team at a large rehabilitation center. Through trial and error, Dale gradually became competent in his chosen profession.

Gaining Insight Through Trial and Error

As an art therapist at a large rehabilitation center, Dale had achieved a certain level of confidence and skill. Years of developing his practice helped him achieve a good reputation from his team members. He was known for his impressive results with depressed patients who had lost some motor functions due to a brain injury. He developed the ability to remain patient even when the fires of impatience raged within him. Dale credited his success with constantly reviewing his skills and giving himself time to question and evaluate his methods as a caregiver. Step by step, he began to understand a discipline of practice that is similar to what Dr. Atul Gawande advocates for healthcare. Through trial and error, Dale was able to discern the best options for treatment. He began to understand the discipline of practice. Through his use of repeated actions, he honed his skills to perfection. In this sense, practice requires us to focus on both personal and professional improvement.

Another meaning of practice has to do with one's professional work or business, such as the practice of a lawyer, physician, or nurse practitioner. In Dale's case, it was the practice of art therapy. Dale's work was a practice wherein each day and each encounter demanded an openness and an attitude of hospitality. The expectation and performance of skills with a spirit of selflessness, and a truthfulness that engendered trust, were the skills Dale developed over time. While most of his clients struggled with the acceptance of being partially paralyzed, drifting in and out of their fears, Dale knew he had to be their moor, their anchor, where they could tether the anguish and hopelessness they felt. Practice took on a different meaning, one that recognized the needs of the patient or client come first, even when one is having a bad hair day. Such was his experience with Bart Morgani, a construction worker in his 60s. One day on the job, Bart felt dizzy, and before he knew it, passed out, only to awaken in the emergency room. Upon diagnosis, it was discovered that he suffered a cerebrovascular accident, commonly called a stroke. He had a history of being overweight, smoked cigarettes, and had high blood pressure.

In the ambulance, Bart started to respond as if in a dream. He woke up and wondered why he was in an ambulance. By the time he arrived in the emergency room, with the staff continuing the protocol for stroke victims, he felt even more confused. Accustomed to self-sufficiency, he tried to get up, wanting to go home, when he realized he could not move his right leg. It seemed stuck to the gurney he was lying on. He didn't realize he also was hooked up to a heart monitor and an intravenous drip. In a daze, Bart looked at the nurse who began to reposition him on the gurney, as he struggled to put words to sounds, he mumbled, "What happened to me?"

Bart spent a few days in the Intensive Care Unit, then went to the Stroke Unit, where he responded well to medications and treatments. In less than a week, he was transferred to a nearby rehabilitation center where he first encountered Dale, only a day after he was admitted. Bart was in a wheelchair in the center's activity room, after finishing a physical therapy session. Dale introduced himself and asked if he could pull a chair over to talk with him. He wanted Bart to know he was a member of the interdisciplinary team and asked if he could do an admitting evaluation. Bart's response was flat and monotoned: "Do what you need to do. I'm not going anywhere." Dale responded, "Mr. Morgani, may I call you Bart? I'd like to do an admitting evaluation, but I sense your frustration in not being able to go anywhere?" "Damn!" Bart interrupted, "Look at me! One day I can run circles around the guys at work, and then the next day I'm in a wheelchair. What the hell can you do for me?" Again, it was not about Dale, but about Bart, as he was struggling to adjust to his new normal.

The challenge was clear, and the invitation was complex. On one hand, the passive invitation to come and do what you need to do, and on the other, the active cry for help. To complicate it more, Bart didn't have a clue how art therapy could help him recover and gain confidence. He didn't know anyone on the job who did art in their spare time. He was a construction worker, a craftsman, rough and tough with guys who had their own lingo and culture. Dale had a flashback just before his graduation from high school, when he had to pick up his father from a construction site. He was taken back by the lingo of his father's coworkers: "Give me the mother fucking hammer, Bill. Do you have all your goddamn tools?" and "Get your ass moving, Joe, it almost quitting time."

"Bart," Dale responded, "We are going to work together, to reactivate those brain cells and neurons that were damaged because of your stroke. But I need your help. There will be days like today, when you feel like, 'What's the use?' There will also be days you will feel a sense of accomplishment because of the hard work you've done. What I can guarantee you is that by working together, we can achieve some goals step by step." That day, Bart and Dale began a journey together that led Bart to discover his latent creativity, which he eventually used to transform both his body and his mind.

Dale learned Bart loved to cook recipes he learned from his Italian grandmother. She told him, "Heaven smells like an Italian kitchen." He talked about the homegrown tomatoes he raised to make spaghetti sauce. Dale asked Bart to imagine walking through the garden: "What was it like?" Bart's eyes glistened as he told Dale about the dinner guests who marveled at the taste of his family's spaghetti sauce. One evening, Bart's cousin, on a visit from Rome, asked about the sauce and who made it. His cousin said it was like the sauce served in the best restaurants in Rome. Bart swelled up like a peacock, smiled, and said, "Si, questa cena e molto buono, ce la farà questa mangare." ("Yes, this dinner is very good. I made it.")

Dale and Bart spent time exploring Bart's Italian heritage, especially some of the masterpieces of Italian art. Bart's wife, Angelina, brought in a scrapbook filled with pictures of their recent trip to Rome, which Dale and Bart examined together. While there are many ways to stimulate the nervous system, to activate neurons and muscle, one look at Michelangelo's David or Bernini's Colonnades of St. Peter's can incite awe and amazement. "Bart," Dale asked, "Remember the first day we met, and you questioned what could art therapy do for you? You are Italian—art is in your blood." Bart discovered art could help him focus, help with his dexterity, uplift his mood, and in some ways, inspire hope for the future. Dale was persistent in helping Bart discover new ways to stimulate his nervous system and mood. It was about practice, day in and day out, and building a trusted relationship with Dale that helped Bart dig deep into his own Soul and continue on the road to recovery. Under the mask of this tough construction worker was a gentle spirit that continually inspired him despite the challenges he faced. After six weeks of intensive therapy, Bart was ready to walk out of the rehab center with a few cracks and fissures in the macho mask he so desperately wore.

The Art of Practice

While one must practice to become more skilled and efficient, practice can also be understood to mean a particular type of work, such as medicine, dentistry, fire prevention, law, or counseling. One can be called a practitioner, like a general practitioner or a nurse practitioner. Another can have a law practice, or a therapy or coaching practice. There is something dynamic in having a practice, as the practice itself, along with the practitioner, is constantly evolving. Thus, we hear about those practicing the art of medicine or being engaged in the healing arts. If we agree that practice is important to master our professional skills and that we, as caregivers, may be involved in a particular practice or occupation, is it possible for us to reimagine the art of caregiving as not only a practice, but a spiritual practice? As discussed in Chapter One, the dance of caregiving involves an interplay between the caregiver, their internal world, and the one receiving the care. During this dance, each party is challenged to create new steps, as the tasks of caregiving lead the caregiver to a deeper understanding of healing and transformation. Similarly, the act of caregiving challenges the one receiving care to be vulnerable, receptive, and hospitable in accepting the care given. Each supports the other like adventurers on a journey of self-discovery. We can speak of many different types of caregiving, and many different recipients of care, but no matter how short or extended the encounter is between the caregiver and the one being served, the opportunity for personal and professional growth is always available.

I believe caregiving is a practice, and as such, can be artfully practiced. The art of caregiving, though not consciously seen or experienced as such, has a spiritual foundation. The art of caregiving may be viewed as a spiritual practice when technical skills are interwoven with compassion and care. What makes the practice of caregiving a spiritual endeavor is that the act of caregiving invites both the caregiver and the one seeking care to listen to the promptings of their Soul. Herein lies the possibility of transformation. The ordinary becomes extraordinary, the work becomes a calling, and the art of caregiving becomes a healing art.

The caregiver is firmly committed to serving, which requires a selflessness to use one's talents and skills to care for those in need. Caregivers also want to build relationships with those seeking their care. We may ask, what motivates us to care? What sustains us in the tasks of caregiving? What is the unique life force or energy that moves us into action? Think of the unique calling that led you to become a caregiver and the values that sustain you as a caregiver. Caregiving is a spiritual practice because each participant is challenged daily to respond to those who are in need, those who suffer, those who are in danger from floods, hurricanes, earthquakes, or wildfires, those who are ill, those who are victims of domestic violence, those who need coaching and mentoring, and those who are elderly and dying. This is a heroic enterprise which requires diligent practice, yet we do it every day. And the response itself is a practice. The "how" and "why" we do what we do is what makes caregiving a spiritual practice.

The Rituals of Practice

Each caregiving profession has its own rituals for receiving new members and sustaining them within the profession. There are codes of conduct, codes of ethics, and various procedures to follow. Remember the safety protocol of the first responders and the firefighters as retold by Allison in Chapter Four? By the time they arrived at the site, the aircraft was engulfed in flames. The possibility of the gas tanks exploding prevented them from risking their lives to save the pilot, whose cabin was already engulfed in flames. Consider the rituals you experience when you want to see your primary physician: making an appointment, checking in upon arrival, and confirming your identity, proof of insurance, and current medications. There is a comparable ritual of triage screening in a busy emergency room, and washing one's hands before and after visiting a patient to prevent the spread of infection is yet another ritual we practice.

Rituals are both exciting and routine, sometimes bordering on pure drudgery. First responders check and replace the stores of emergency drugs and equipment after each run. Nurses check and recheck the "crash" cart used for "code blues" (a code indicating someone needs CPR) on the hospital floors. After each fire, firefighters clean and reroll fire hoses, as well as prepare the truck for the next emergency. These rituals have helped develop the best practices in each profession. We are familiar with the safety regulations when we fly, the protocols for first responders, or some of the different protocols and best practices in medicine. It was Captain "Sully" Sullenberger's ritual of reviewing the checklist with his crew that saved all aboard his flight when the engines failed and forced him to land the plane in the Hudson River. The crew was well prepared for such an emergency.

Ritual Practices within Spiritual Traditions

Consider the ritual practices of the many spiritual traditions, where a practice is a form of discipline such as meditation, yoga, ritual prayers, singing, or chanting. Each practice begins with a unique intention or goal which requires a firm sense of purpose, strength of will, and determination. The dancing of the whirling dervishes of the Sufi Islamic tradition is one such spiritual practice, which seeks union with the transcendent, the Holy Other, the Divine. Dancing becomes the ritual and the discipline. The different practices of meditation, the reading of Sacred Scriptures from many spiritual traditions, or the use of rosary beads or knotted threads to count prayers in the Buddhist, Catholic, Hindu, and Islamic traditions are other examples of a spiritual practice where repetition and concentration lead one to a deeper meditative and prayerful state.

Ancient healing practices acknowledged discipline as necessary in providing treatment and healing remedies. The Hippocratic Oath and ethical codes of practice establish principles many caregivers still follow today. Caring for those in need of our care is an integral part of many spiritual and religious traditions. Thomas Moore said, "The very essence of spirituality is to tend to physical and emotional illnesses."[125] Seeking balance and integration of body and Soul are reflected in the Chinese notion of yin and yang, symbolized by an image in which each half contains a bit of its opposite. Jewish healing practices stress being right with God, the creator and healer, as well as following the principles of the Torah in discovering the Kabbalistic wisdom to promote health and treat disease. In the Christian tradition, the Gospel mandates of Matthew to care for the least members of a community are known and practiced as the corporal works of mercy. Islamic healing practices promote practical intervention strategies within an Islamic-based theoretical framework which outlines the four major elements of the human being. These practices include cognitive restructuring using the Qur'an and traditions of Prophet Muhammad (PBUH), spiritual remedies presented through the repetition of prescribed prayers, invoking blessings upon the Prophet, and reflecting upon a behavioral log of daily actions.[126] Recall the ritual washing the family of their mother requested mentioned in Chapter Eight.

Less Profound Rituals

Other rituals are as simple as brushing your teeth, walking your dog, going on a run, or exercising at the gym. Our routine manner of preparing meals is another kind of ritual. Some of us like to have a lite supper. Others prefer to make dinner their most substantia! meal of the day. Each of us has a different way of slowing down in the evening, using rituals such as reading, spending time with family, watching an old movie, or listening to classical music, while others simply "crash" after a stressful day. We might take a favorite route on our way to work, and as caregivers, we prepare for work as best we can. Caregivers are also ready, even hypervigilant, to drop everything for an emergent situation. How many times have we heard the phrase, "My day is not going as planned"—as if we could predict the future!

Rituals engage us in life and its daily routines. Caregivers are trained to follow procedures and protocols which define how we will respond to a particular situation. As such, may we also use the word "ritual" to describe a protocol? Are protocols not the same as rituals, in that they are both a designated way of performing a task? The outcomes, of course, are the intended goals of the intervention in meeting the needs of those served. The meeting between caregiver and the one served becomes an opportunity for healing and transformation. In the relationship that is formed, each is sustained in the act of giving and receiving. The following story of Elliot and Benjamin relates how two semi-estranged twins came together and rediscovered their spiritual bond through the dance of caregiving.

"Mrs. Jones, I think there is someone else up there."

From their earliest memories, Elliot and Benjamin had a desire to support and care for each other. They were fraternal twins, who at the request of their father, were encouraged to be independent and "not like other twins." A paradox indeed. Each had their own group of friends and attended different high schools; one travelled to the west coast, and the other remained near home. Their arrival into the world was even more of a surprise: six weeks before their mother's due date, the water in which they inhabited seemed to disappear. Elliot, the more rambunctious of the two, arrived first, weighing just under three pounds. Everything seemed to be in order until, to the amazement of their mother and everyone else in the room, the doctor pronounced incredulously: "I think there is someone else up there!" And of course, there was: Elliot's twin brother, Benjamin arrived, weighing just over three pounds. They often joked their mother never got over the surprise.

Sixty-five years later, Benjamin was admitted to the hospital suffering from COPD, or Chronic Obstructive Pulmonary Disease. His wife had died two years earlier and they had no children. While Elliot and Benjamin had visited with each other throughout the years, they never had the opportunity to explore and discuss their respective life paths with each other. Elliot, who was divorced and lived alone, was shocked when he heard about Benjamin's poor prognosis. Benny, as he liked to be called, could no longer live on his own, and before either of them could ask for help or offer an invitation, Benny said, "I just want to go home." "Of course, you do," Elliot said, "I want you to come home with me." Their embrace knocked the air out of each of them. Being twins, they knew their love for each other would make their journey of caregiving easier. The doctors did not give Benny a good prognosis and told him he had six to twelve months to live. Elliot was determined to make sure his twin brother didn't die alone. Soon enough, Benny was stable enough to be discharged.

Neither brother was prepared for the tasks of caregiving, nor were they prepared for the demands of coping with COPD. The visiting nurse set up a program for Benny and was always a call away. Some days were better for Benny, some days were better for

Elliot, some days were good for them both and some days were, in a manner of speaking, pretty bad for each of them. Benny's task was to change his perspective: he needed to stop being a powerless victim and learn to welcome the gifts life was giving him. This rubbed against the grain, as everything within Benny screamed for independence. Independence and self-reliance are different than being a victim, but welcoming the gift of caregiving from another is an act of great courage. Elliot, on the other hand, struggled with his impatience and wished Benny would do more, even though he knew the severity of Benny's diagnosis.

Elliot's task was to deal with the tension between simultaneously being Benny's twin brother and his primary caregiver. At home, Benny needed complete care: assistance to the bathroom, shower, and dressing. While Benny struggled with asking for help, Elliot struggled with being the caregiver Benny needed. Despite Elliot's experience as a registered nurse, who technically knew what needed to be done, the emotional attachment to his brother created a different kind of caregiving relationship. It was difficult to see Benny in his current condition, and it was even difficult to know his brother's life expectancy was limited. In a way, after all these years, when the opportunity came to spend time with his twin brother, Elliot was confronted with what he initially thought was a missed opportunity. He decided to keep his feelings to himself and put them on a back burner, not realizing his very intention was still being unconsciously processed.

About two weeks after Benny was discharged from the hospital, as Elliot and Benny were finishing breakfast, Benny remarked "Well these days have been quite a workout for the both of us, haven't they? Do you remember several years ago when we both went on the men's retreat?" Elliot nodded his head in agreement with a big Cheshire cat grin, "Sure do!" Benny continued "I remember the talking stick, a stick which was passed around in the circle for each person to speak. Each had to be respectful and listen to what the other person was saying with no commentary or interruptions. Elliott, can we do this now? We don't have a talking stick, but the wooden spoon over by the stove should do. I want to share a few thoughts. I want to be as honest as I can, and I want you to listen. Then, I want you to be as honest as you can while I listen." Elliot rose to get the wooden spoon and passed it over to Benny. "I, too, have been waiting for this moment, now that we are sort of settled," replied Elliot. "You have the spoon. Go for it."

Benny then took the deepest breath he could and hoped Elliot would not be embarrassed by what he was going to say: "You know Elliot, I have always been a crusty old barnacle, always holding in my feelings and keeping what I was thinking close to my chest. I don't know if I can find the right words but thank you. Thank you for taking me in and loving me as your brother." Tears began to flow from Benny's eyes as he continued, "I'm a mess, and as much as I want to do everything for myself, I can't. This just pisses me off. I have always been independent, in control, and now I can't even go to the bathroom without your help. I know yesterday when I nearly fell, I was careless, focused on getting there quickly instead of watching where I was going and asking for your help. Please forgive me for being such a burden. I hate being so vulnerable, every fiber of my manhood rebels against it, and yet, if I am truly going to love you, I must accept your gracious gift of caregiving. I must accept you."

Elliot spontaneously reached out his hands across the breakfast table to meet those of Benny. In the silence of the embrace, they felt what they both had prayed for during their years of separation. The squeeze of their clasped hands seemed to melt away the years, and in this present moment, time stopped, and they each experienced being a brother to each other.

What seemed like a moment lasted about five minutes, as they stared at each other with tears running down their flushed faces, tenderly holding each other's hands. Elliot then responded, "I guess I broke the rules, as I usually do, in reaching out to you. I wasn't sure if you were finished but I couldn't help myself." Benny agreed he was finished and passed the wooden spoon over to Elliot. Arms folded, Elliot sat back in his chair and began: "I've always had difficulty in putting my feelings into words, you know me. But when I heard about your diagnosis and learned you'd have to sell your home and go to a nursing facility, something in me realized how much I have missed you, and how much I wanted you to spend the remaining years of life with me. You know I am divorced, and my two sons live on the west coast. I know they would be thrilled to know you are here. You are their only uncle."

Elliot took a sip of water and knew what he was going to say would be difficult. "Benny, I know the visiting nurses and aids have been very helpful, but I must confess, I had no idea what caregiving was about. I had no idea how the 24/7 responsibility would affect me. I cringe at the site of blood, let alone be responsible to help you the way I have been doing. I didn't know I had the strength. But I am learning, digging deep within me for those values I hold the most, and I am realizing I would not want it any other way. Just as it is difficult for you to submit to receiving care, so is it difficult for me to be your caregiver. I am learning the danger or shadow side of being a caregiver. Our relationship can be uneven. I'm the one in charge, sort of like nurse Ratchet, and you are the one who has to listen. This is not what being a caregiver to you means to me. Don't get me wrong, caring for you is having an effect on me. I have to deal with my own shit, stuff I've burying for years. Now it just pops up, almost laughing at me, wondering if I have the courage needed to confront these fear gremlins and shoo them off. A few days ago, I thought I was going to care for you and that it would be a one-way street. Somehow in the bond we are sharing this morning, I have come to believe you are helping me be a better man." Benny knew how difficult it was for Elliot to be as vulnerable as he was, always making a big deal that he was the older twin (older by only four minutes!).

As the weeks grew into months, and months into years, again at another routine debriefing, Elliot remarked, "Benny, do you remember what your doctor said three years ago—that you only have twelve to eighteen months to live? You are out living him by a year and a half." They both chuckled. As their visiting nurse, I witnessed how the bond of love they shared actually effected Benny's condition. His symptoms decreased to such an extent that he was able to travel to Elliot's grandson's bar mitzvah in Los Angeles. For Elliot, caregiving was initially a chore, but over time it became a daily spiritual practice, fed by a river of unending brotherhood. Benny's struggle became moot against Elliot's desire to care, even though he felt awkward and inexperienced. Caregiving became a journey, a pilgrimage of sorts, as the archetypal energies guided and supported them. In their own way, they each found the will and the courage to discover the healer function within themselves and in one another.

Elliot and Benny's experience is something we, as caregivers, can identify with and recognize. The brothers were hesitant to be vulnerable with each other, while at the same time, there was a desire to do so. How often do we, as caregivers, feel this way with our peers and team members? Although not always fully able to articulate what they were experiencing, Elliott and Benny recognized their limitations, and their journey was grounded in the archetype of the Wounded Healer. The nature of the Wounded Healer necessitates both an interplay and relationship between the caregiver and the one cared for that develops trust, commitment, and companionship.

Caregiving becomes a crucible of Soul-making within which the caregiver discovers depth, value, heart, and personal meaning. Similarly, those who need care must trust their intuition. According to Thomas Moore, "Even very sick or burdened people have remarkable spirits, including creativity, the capacity to cope with illness and mortality, and the wonderfully human drive to find one's own life's meaning." The journey becomes one of pilgrimage, as archetypal energies guide and support us. As caregivers, our journey is one of both personal and professional growth, and its path can span a lifetime.

Caregiving as a Pilgrimage

I want to introduce you to another perspective of caregiving, that of pilgrimage. Pilgrimage leads one to mystery and to one's sacred path, such as what led us into the profession of caregiving and what continues to sustain us. A pilgrimage is inherently spiritual and leads one to Soul. We may have read Chaucer's *Canterbury Tales* in high school, or are familiar with pilgrimages to sacred sites as described in literature, art, and mythology. There are many sacred paths and "sacred ways" that mark the world's temples and shrines, such as those at Delphi, Delos, Jerusalem, Mecca, Santiago de Compostela, and Lourdes. I consider caregiving a sacred path, a unique pilgrimage, where the caregiver and the one seeking care journey together. Their journey challenges them to be faithful to their commitment to each other which could lead them to a deeper sense of themselves, as if coming home again, as experienced by Elliott and Benny.

Why Do People Go?

In *The Archetype of Pilgrimage: Outer Action with Inner Meaning*, Jean and Wallace Clift list fifteen reasons for making a pilgrimage. Many of them are applicable to those who are caregivers and those who are in need of care, such as: to draw near to something sacred within themselves, to have the opportunity to seek pardon and reconciliation, to hope when hope seems elusive, to ask for a miracle, to give thanks, to express gratitude to the Divine, to answer an inner call to go, to regain lost or forgotten parts of one's life, to honor a vow, and to prepare for death.[127] Here lies the thesis of this work: caregiving is a pilgrimage, a sacred place where caregivers come to experience the transcendent nature of their work and in doing so are healed and transformed. In short, caregiving is a spiritual practice.

Wholeness and a renewed understanding of oneself can be borne out of the joys and trials of caregiving. The cycle of descent, journeying, and returning is completed, and the wisdom gained from the experience becomes transformative. Pilgrimage is also etched in the hearts of those seeking healing, who venture mythically on the path to wholeness. Crossing a threshold into an experience of pilgrimage marks one, not only physically, but also soulfully. Christian theologian Richard Niebuhr wrote, "What we apprehend outwardly becomes part of the lasting geography of our Souls; the pilgrim in us begins to awaken."[128]

The nurse, physician, counselor, pastor, spiritual leader, coach, first responder, emergency medical responder, safety officer, firefighter, educator, and mentor know that the geography of their Souls leads them to excel as caregivers. Pilgrims mark their journeys in the soil of the sacred paths they create with their sweat, tears, and blood. The caregivers and those they care for do the same in the patient, long suffering that each may experience. Life has its way of giving us our share of painful experiences as caregivers.

Thresholds are crossed during preparations, leave-taking, and new beginnings, as well as during participation in the spirituality of the pilgrimage itself. A pilgrimage is both a physical and symbolic act in which each pilgrim seeks to transform their journey into an active and dynamic event. According to Jungian analyst Robert A. Johnson, pilgrimage "becomes a symbol-in-motion that carries the power of the inner world into visible and physical form."[129] As caregivers, are we aware of how the invisible world, our Soul, speaks to us? What do we long for as a caregiver? Our caregiving can be both a symbolic journey and an archetypal pilgrimage which renders the power of the inner world visible between the caregiver and the one being served. According to Campbell, the pilgrimage of healing "is symbolical of that divine creative and redemptive image, which is hidden within all of us, only waiting to be known and rendered into life."[130]

In answering an inner call to participate in such a journey, the one who needs caregiving, as well as the caregiver, discovers that the path they have chosen leads them to a greater understanding of each other and to personal transformation.

The journey becomes a path marked by many, often unplanned, crossings of thresholds which define it. Caregivers become the facilitators and the tour guides, assisting those embarking with them on the journey to healing. It can come as a surprise to caregivers that as tour guides, they too become pilgrims. A good tour guide facilitates the traveler's arrival to a moment of discovery and then stands back; a bad tour guide talks too much and spoils the moment by babbling about his own experiences. The good tour guide listens for clues to where the traveler might like to go next; the bad one has a set itinerary primarily designed for his own convenience. The good tour guide is widely travelled and delights in opportunities to serve a diversity of clients; the bad one is fearful and disparaging of "foreigners." The bad tour guide becomes hysterical when plans go awry and an unforeseen detour is required; the good one reframes this change as an adventure, as fodder for a great story of how trouble was overcome, the problem understood, an insight learned, a transformation made possible.

As you have been warned many times already, the practice of caregiving is not for everyone. There are trials, rabbit holes to fall into and the dangers of not caring for oneself; there is the shadow side of caregiving, which often involves compassion fatigue and burnout. We began with the importance of practice, then explored how we, as caregivers, may have a practice. We explored the patience of Dale as an art therapist and were drawn into the story of Elliot and Benjamin. Finally, we concluded with the realization that we, as caregivers, are pilgrims on life's journey. The concluding chapter, "Warning: Our Tank is Almost Empty," will explore the symptoms and the causes of compassion fatigue and burnout. We will discover that because we care, because we give compassionate care, we are naturally prone to fatigue and exhaustion. Because we care, we may be prone to compassion fatigue and her two sisters: burnout, and secondary traumatic stress. These are common experiences of caregivers and should not be considered extraordinary or abnormal. At some point in their career, many caregivers experience compassion fatigue. Building compassion resilience by rediscovering interior strengths is what guides caregivers through the storms of caregiving.

A Moment of Reflection

Time for another stop on the journey. Take your time to reflect on the questions below. Again, this is not a test, no perfect scores, you are a winner just the way you are.

1. Was there a moment during this chapter when you could identify with your own journey as a caregiver?

2. Is identifying caregiving as a spiritual practice new for you? In light of the previous chapter on spirituality, can you give an example of how you were empowered as a caregiver?

3. Were the stories of Dale and Bart and Elliot and Benny compelling to you? In what ways?

_____

_____

_____

_____

_____

_____

_____

_____

_____

_____

_____

_____

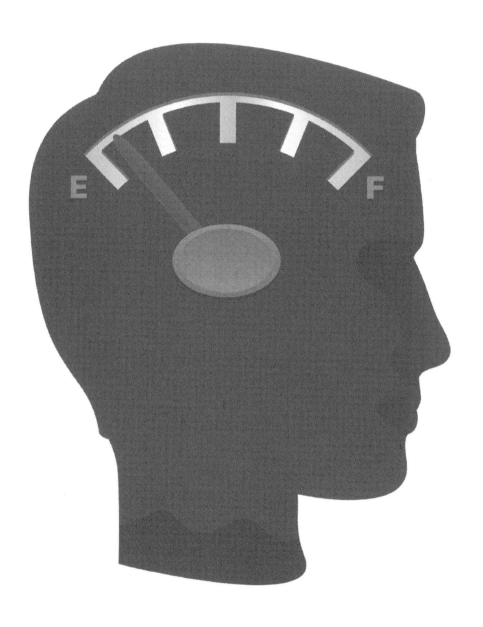

Chapter 10 - Warning: Our Tank is Almost Empty

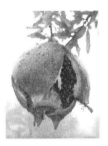

We have within us the human capacity to push forward even when it hurts. Amid confusion, exhaustion, and stress, we know we will find the interior strength to forge ahead, find the necessary fuel, take a short reprieve, and carry on. We, as caregivers, have had many experiences of just sucking it up and continue relying (hopefully) on our reserve. A little bit of pressure here, a little bit there, always believing we can go on until we can't. We forge ahead, often unaware that our tank is almost empty. Sputter, sputter, until one extra shift, one more trauma, one more instance of stuffing our feelings, and until we're forced to pull over on the side of the road. We have just enough left to cry out for help. Finally, we realize our tank is almost empty.

What happens when we are unable to hear, let alone listen to, the inner promptings of our Soul trying to warn us? Why have these warning signs fallen on deaf ears? Have we neglected them for so long we've become numb to them? Maybe we are simply not conscious enough of the effect secondary traumatic stress has had on us. We run out of our reserve, and for a moment we feel paralyzed, overcome with emotion, overcome with what to do, overcome with fear that no one will listen or understand.

My natural inclination to show compassion for others led to my experience of compassion fatigue, which included elements of secondary traumatic stress and burnout. When I came to this screeching halt over twenty-five years ago, my colleagues wondered why I couldn't keep up, and they simply did not understand, which only led to a heightened sense of abandonment. On the outside, I didn't show any signs of fatigue. Internally, I felt emotionally hypersensitive, like a million neurons going off which needed to be corralled. At times, I felt overwhelmed; at other times, emotionally flat, and still other times oversensitive with a short fuse as I was unable to defend myself.

What I was experiencing may have reminded my colleagues on an unconscious level of what they, too, may have been experiencing. I just remember how much I needed them to understand and, at the same time, how much they didn't. I knew if I had been in a terrible accident or injured at work, they would have understood. I imagined myself in a hospital bed with casts on, my broken leg pinned and raised up in a sling. But the train wreck I was experiencing resulted from a lack of support and a lack of self-care which could have addressed my physical, psychological, interpersonal, and spiritual needs. I was just too busy to consider them. There were, however, faint revelations that something was wrong, as I was becoming increasingly exhausted. Burnout is a state of fatigue or frustration brought about by devotion to a cause, way of life, or a particular relationship that fails to produce an expected reward.[131]

I won the trifecta, as I experienced all three of these. I certainly had a passion and devotion to a cause. I supported the mission of the non-profit I was working with, and finally, when building a relationship with my two co-facilitators, it always seemed to be two against one. I was the lone man standing and often found myself in an unhealthy relationship triangle. Recall the words of Patricia Smith quoted earlier: "In order to experience a sense of peace, well-being and belonging in our world, we must learn to integrate the following into our lives: a source of strength other than ourselves, a tradition of prayer, meditation, or worship that allows us to disengage from the everyday world, and a practice of rituals that have the power to restore calmness, serenity, continuity and hope to our lives."[132] At one time or another in my life, each of these practices had been present, but somehow, at some point, I got lost.

My well was dry or, to use another metaphor, I was bankrupt. The symptoms, like the arms of compassion fatigue leading to burnout, had ensnared me. There was, however, enough reserve left to make the decision to visit a friend, Leo, who was a pastoral counselor. I remembered his compassion when, a year or so previously, he invited me to come and chat if I ever needed help. It is important for caregivers to respond with compassion when we experience our teammates reaching out for help. His compassion seared through any resistance I had in seeking help. His compassion was the reason I was drawn to choose him. From a coaching or counseling perspective, this was about building a therapeutic and trusting relationship.

Leo was most generous in making time to see me. We set up a schedule for my visits three times a week. I didn't realize how much I needed his arms of compassion to keep me falling off a cliff of despair. He introduced me to the terms compassion fatigue and burnout, which were new concepts for me. After a month, I remember asking him how much longer it will take for me to get back on my feet. I had taken a leave of absence and was about to apply for the company's disability. At this moment, I felt my recovery was going to take more time and effort than I expected. I wanted to know more about burnout, so I asked Leo, "On a scale of one to ten, how serious do you feel my experience of burnout is?" Leo responded truthfully: on a scale from 1 to 10, he felt the degree of my burnout was between 8 and 9; he considered 10 to be irreversible.

I was numbed by his words. He asked me how long I had been in this conflicted situation of wearing myself out. "Three years," I responded. Then Leo said, "It will take you three years to recover. One day you will find you crossed over the bridge, and you will know the difference. You are bankrupt and have to restore your energy, to pay off the debt. You know, burnout is a physical and emotional exhaustion which is caused by stress. This type of stress leads to disillusionment and depression."

I remember asking Leo, still hanging on to a remnant of my past behaviors, that I wanted to do what was best for me and what the Holy Spirit wanted of me. I laugh now at his response. He calmly responded, "When you feel the most conflicted or overwhelmed, do what is the easiest. I want to repeat this. It is important for you to choose what is the easiest choice when you feel overwhelmed when many choices race through your consciousness. This is what the Holy Spirit is asking of you." The words did sink in, and I attribute them to helping me recover. Imagine, do what is the easiest in a world of getting it done yesterday! That was over twenty-five years ago. So, what's in a name? When you hear the words compassion fatigue, burnout, and secondary traumatic stress, what do they mean?

What's in a Name?

Before we explore the history, research, symptoms, treatment, and experience of compassion fatigue, I'd like to begin by examining the words "compassion" and "fatigue." What is in a name? Seems from the get-go, compassion fatigue is a state of exhaustion. We, as caregivers, experience vicarious trauma due to our practice of compassion in the work we do. (Recall our earlier discussion of the wounded healer in Chapter Six, "Love is a Wounded Healer.")

"What's in a Name?" Juliet asks Romeo in William Shakespeare's Romeo and Juliet. A name identifies, as well as reveals a hidden meaning. Parzival, when asked his name by his cousin Signue, responds in French: "Bon fiz, cher fiz, bea fiz—that's what they used to call me, those who knew me at home."[133] There was a hidden meaning to his name, which means "Pierce-through-the-heart" or, said another way, a person who endures suffering.[134]

The same can be said about compassion fatigue. It is all in its name: compassion, good; fatigue, not so good. No time to admit any sign of weakness or fatigue. (God forbid we need to take a few days off here or there!) We, as caregivers, understand the demands compassion has on us. To enter the world of the one who needs care is to enter a world of potential suffering, unanswered questions, doubts, fears, and pain. It means to suffer with them. Hence the meaning of the word compassion, from the Latin root *com*, meaning "with" or "together," and *passion*, meaning "to suffer." It is important to emphasize that compassion fatigue is not something extraordinary, nor is it a mental illness designated for an unlucky few. Compassion fatigue occurs because caregivers care. Let me repeat this: *Compassion fatigue occurs because caregivers care.* It is an inevitable side effect of being a caregiver.

Psychotherapist Charles Figley begins his book about compassion fatigue with these words: "There is a cost to caring. Professionals who listen to clients' stories of fear, pain, and suffering may feel similar fears, pains, and sufferings because they care."[135] The question then becomes, how do caregivers deal with the fatigue which is, in some sense, to be expected? How do they prevent the extreme symptoms of fatigue and exhaustion and build up resilience? Compassion defines who we are. It is the tonic that refreshes humankind. But even though we perform this sacred work, we are not gods. We can and do run out of energy, which needs to be replaced. There is an interior discipline and resilience we must create to address the gremlins lurking about us.

Beyond Expectations

Jean, a seasoned intensive care (ICU) nurse, was caring for a patient named Mr. Lin. He was admitted the day before from the ER after suffering a cerebral vascular accident (CVA) at home. After a family conference with the doctor, it was determined that there was little chance of his recovery due to the massive bleed he had the day before. The family agreed to make him a "no code" and a do not resuscitate (DNR) order was put in place.

The family asked Jean if they could dress Mr. Lin in his tuxedo before he died. Although it initially seemed like an unusual request, Jean surmised there was more to the story. Mr. Linn and his family were devout Buddhists, and Jean knew the family had already called their priests to come and recite ritual prayers for Mr. Linn as he died.

Jean asked the family about their request to dress Mr. Linn in a tuxedo, and their response was simple and direct: "We want him to look good when he meets his relatives." Jean may have considered her sensitivity and compassion toward Mr. Lin's family to be routine, but as she told me this story, I recognized her compassionate care went beyond expectations. At first, the family's request seemed somewhat unusual, but Jean listened to their needs, created a hospitable environment for the family, and demonstrated excellent compassionate care.

The Discipline of Compassion

Although most would agree that compassion is a value to be lived, its practice is often difficult in a culture that values competition and individualism. Gawande suggested selflessness, the art of accepting responsibility for the other and placing those needs ahead of oneself, is necessary and demands an interior discipline.[136] Self-care is not being selfish but is the discipline or guardrails that channel compassion. Another word for discipline might be temperance, the ability to temper and guide one's energy in making soulful decisions. There are multifaceted expressions of compassion, somewhat like the different levels of hospitality discussed in Chapter Five. The three aspects of compassion focus on: the caregiver and his or her response to the one in need, the interchange between the caregiver and the one seeking care, and the compassion the caregiver needs to listen to the interior promptings of their Soul. Does the caregiver hear the cry of the one in need? Does the one in need have a story to tell and needs a compassionate ear? Finally, does the caregiver take the risk, showing self-compassion in exploring what the stirrings their Soul wish to articulate?

Nouwen et al. argued compassion is more than a general kindness or tenderheartedness: "Compassion asks us to go where it hurts, to enter into places of pain, to share in brokenness, fear, confusion and anguish."[137] Listen to how these words resonate with an invitation to understand the story of the one seeking care, and most importantly, how these actions resonate within our Souls. The authors continued, "Compassion requires us to cry out with those in misery, to mourn with those who are lonely, to weep with those in tears. Compassion requires us to be weak with those who are weak, to be vulnerable with the vulnerable, powerless with those who are powerless. Compassion means full immersion in the condition of being human."

Notice the compelling demand of the caregiver to reach out and understand the story of the one in need as a member of the community and thus support community efforts in the alleviation of social issues. On the other hand, there is a subtle, almost hidden invitation to allow one to recognize these feelings within oneself. Yes, there are times we experience loneliness; we feel the need to cry, and we feel weak and vulnerable. Sometimes when we appear strong, we feel powerless. In the condition of being human, we, as caregivers, share what all caregivers experience around the world, namely the universal practice of compassion in our work.

We care, and this is the starting point of all that we do as caregivers. No matter how objective we believe we are, we experience the trauma, the pain, and the suffering of those we care for, even when we struggle to remain emotionally detached. Because we care, sometimes we get exhausted, and sometimes we need help to carry the burden of emotional, physical, and psycho-spiritual experiences we carry. The cords that tie us up with the misconception that we must do it all ourselves need to be loosened, and better to be loosened by our own methods and practice. It is better to make a connection with a family member, friend, colleague, or pastoral counselor than to have these cords cut in an emergent situation. Dr. Eric Gentry suggested that when we empower one or two people who know us well and care about us, we create a compassion resiliency safety net. Choose those who are strong enough to withstand any deflection when we become symptomatic or when we become consistently divergent from the ways we normally act.[138] No matter where we start, no matter what our unique philosophy or spiritual tradition may be, compassion is known and practiced around the world. Who do you know, or rather, who are you drawn to because of their compassion? This was what drew me to Leo. I knew he cared, and in caring he saved my life.

The Universality of Compassion

Compassion is held in high regard and is ranked among the greatest human virtues by every major religious tradition. The practice of compassion is implied in the Golden Rule, which paraphrases Matthew 7:12: "Do to others what you would have them do to you." The Oxford Centre for Interfaith Studies highlights this Golden Rule as part of the Declaration of a Global Ethic. This was formulated by Hans Küng and Karl-Josef Kuschel at the Parliament of the World's

Religions held in Chicago in 1993.[139] Some examples from this declaration are described below.

Within the Hindu tradition, a verse from the Mahabharata articulates the Golden Rule: "This is the sum of duty: do naught unto others which would cause you pain if done to you" (XIII, 114). Compassion is called *daya*, and along with charity and self-control, is one of the three central virtues of the Hindu Tradition.[140] In the Jewish tradition, God is the Compassionate Holy Other and is invoked as the Father of Compassion, suggested Khen Lampert. The words of Leviticus articulate how the compassion of God is lived out in daily life: "You shall love your neighbor as yourself (19:18).[141]

Foremost among God's attributes in the Islamic tradition are mercy and compassion. Every prayer and significant action begins with the invocation of God the Merciful and Compassionate. The Golden Rule is articulated in An-Nawawi 40, Hadith 13 of the Islamic tradition: "No one of you is a believer until he desires for his brother that which he desires for himself."[142] Native American traditions articulate the belief that the foundation of spirituality is respect for life. This belief is reflected in The Iroquois Great Law of Peace, whose first principle states that all people must treat each other fairly. The democratic ideals of this charter inspired Benjamin Franklin, James Madison, and other framers of the U.S. Constitution in their writing of the Constitution and the Bill of Rights.[143]

The sacred scriptures of Sikhism, the Guru Granth Sahib, contain many angs (sayings) of the 16th century Guru Arjan Dev Ji, who gives a Sikh perspective of the Golden Rule: "Do not create enmity with anyone as God is within everyone" (Singh 258). The sacred writings of Confucianism suggest: "Do not do to others what you would not want them to do to you" (Analects of Confucius 15, 25).

Lorne Lander defined compassion in the Buddhist tradition as "a state of mind or heart. Buddhism defines compassion as a mental state of wishing that others may be free from suffering."[144] In the Samyutta Nikaya V, it is written: "A state which is not pleasant or enjoyable for me will not be for another; and how can I impose on another a state which is not enjoyable to me. Compassion is closely related to love, which Buddhism defines as "cherishing others, feeling a sense of closeness with and affection for them."[145] H. H. the Dalai Lama stated the whole purpose of religion is to facilitate love and compassion, patience, tolerance, humility, and forgiveness. Suffering is the part of being human in which one's Soul pain cries out to be heard, understood, and relieved. The call of entering the landscape of pain for the caregiver and the one who seeks help, is not an easy task.

Compassion requires an inner discipline of heroic proportions, grounded in a spirituality that requires a universal perspective. Catholic theologian Henri J. M. Nouwen stated, "Compassion requires us to be weak with those who are weak, to be vulnerable with the vulnerable, powerless with those who are powerless. Compassion means full immersion in the condition of being human."[146]

When a Light Bulb Goes On

Every teacher and professor I know has at least one favorite story about a student experiencing a sudden insight, those special moments when a light bulb goes on. They witness the face of the student brighten as if their neurons just lit up (imagine a cartoon light bulb floating above their head). Such was the experience of Dr. Nathan Edwards, an art professor at a local community college.

One rainy day, during a semester break, Nathan was reminiscing about the previous semester. He had just finished a printmaking class, handed in his grades, and was reviewing printed copies of his students' projects. He reflected on the different encounters he had with his students, who came from a variety of cultural backgrounds and age groups.

As most teachers do, he wondered about their futures as artists, those who were struggling to find themselves, those who did well, and those who simply needed an extra elective and were not interested in art. Then he wondered about those students who not only did well in class, but excelled in their work and had a passion for building a career as artists. Nathan knew, along with many of his colleagues, that it was necessary to have a kind and caring heart for the students he taught. He knew it was not about him, but about a student applying the material in such a way that it made a difference in their life.

One such student was Alexander, whose enthusiasm and motivation in class marked his determination to become a graphic artist. Early in the semester, Alex stayed after class to speak with Nathan. They talked about the class, and the different skills required to be a graphic artist, and the importance of finding professors who could mentor him as his education continued. Then, Alex mentioned how impressed and inspired he was by Nathan's class. Nathan responded, "Yes, I saw your enthusiasm as I was lecturing, and I'm pleased you understood the lesson."

Alexander shared he wanted to be a graphic artist and was particularly interested in Nathan's understanding of and approach to the art of printmaking. Alex's enthusiasm and passion were obvious: not only were his art projects completed on time, but he often created an additional project which continued and developed the theme of the first piece. As the semester continued, Alex stayed after class to help Nathan pack up supplies. On one such afternoon, remembering Nathan's words about the importance of finding the best mentors, Alex asked Nathan if he would be his mentor.

Teachers are generally protective of their time outside the classroom, but this time the invitation to be a mentor resonated with Nathan. He paused and asked if he could share a story with Alex before he gave his answer. Then, Nathan described that one of his art professors in college became a mentor to him, and he explained what it meant to him as a young aspiring artist. Nathan's professor wanted his students to meet other nationally recognized artists. He planned a field trip to visit with an artist who had been a mentor to him. Nathan recalled how the class came to his professor's mentor's studio; they sat on the floor and listened to the artist talk about his work and his love of art.

"Somehow," Nathan continued, "like a flash of lightning, I knew I wanted to be an artist. You see, Alex, that's the responsibility a mentor feels. It's almost like being a high priest in the temple of art, to welcome one into the sanctuary. And that is how I feel about you.

I recognize the same spark I felt when I was your age. Yes, of course, I will be your mentor."

Nathan and Alex continued to meet every week until the class ended. Nathan also hired Alex as a studio assistant. They established a mentor relationship which continued for many years. During Alex's undergraduate and graduate studies, Alex would call or visit Nathan whenever he had a question about an art project. Alex's skills developed, and he was hired by a graphic design company in New York. His work even appeared on the cover of a leading magazine. Nathan was gratified that the hours spent with Alex helped him become an accomplished artist. Proud as a peacock, Nathan invited him back to the college to speak to his students.

Nathan never doubted his decision to mentor Alex, especially since they both came from families who considered art to be a pastime and not a career. Nathan was sensitive to this lack of encouragement, which motivated him to be a mentor. For Nathan, being Alex's mentor was indeed a great reward. If this was not reward enough, Alex invited Nathan to host an art exhibition of their works together in New York. This was the gift they gave each other: the original spark, the lightbulb that clicked on, became the guiding motivation for a friendship that still endures. The art of being a mentor entails helping another find their wings, discover more about themselves as they pursue their passion, and eventually take off and fly on their own. In the story of Nathan and Alex, however, the unexpected reward, was that the duo become peers and colleagues. Nathan reached out in compassion, remembering the compassion shown him by one of his art professors, and in doing so, he created space to understand the story of Alex. He discovered those interior stirrings within himself. The gift of caregiving is that the one who reaches out to serve one in need becomes the one who is transformed and healed.

Symptoms Keep Knocking at the Door

The words of Dave Edmunds song "I hear you knocking, but you can't come in" sum up the tension and the dance of caregiving caregivers often experience. Something in us hears the faint knocking at the door of our consciousness, yet we choose to ignore it. Maybe our knocks are on life support; maybe we are even dead to any awareness that the knocking continues. But like it or not, the Soul is persistent in guiding us toward healing and transformation.

I am reminded of the carved inscription on the lintel over the main door of Jung's house, a quote he borrowed from the Oracle at Delphi: "Vocatus atque non vocatus Deus aderit" which means "Summoned or not summoned, God will be present."[147] Summoned or not summoned, our Soul will guide us. What keeps us from opening the door and saying, "Come in?" What prevents us from creating the space within us to listen, to discern, and to take action? Is it the fear of what we may discover, or is there a fear of feeling vulnerable and a fear of being shamed because we are not professional enough? Is it the fear we will be blamed, even though studies show it is not a flaw within the individual, but rather a systemic flaw in the organization?[148]

I recently spoke with a physician who is the medical director of a large neonatal intensive care unit in the Midwest. In our conversation, she acknowledged that admitting any type of vulnerability among her peers is considered not only a weakness, but a sign of being an incompetent caregiver. Do fears of judgment drown out these interior stirrings of our Soul? Do we use busyness as an excuse to avoid inner exploration? Perhaps we know, on some level, that taking the time to pause will require us to face our fears of acknowledging and tending to our Soul pain. The task for the caregiver is to acknowledge the knocking, open the door, and gently introduce oneself to what needs to be addressed. Easier said than done.

So, What is Fatigue?

Returning to our metaphor of "What is in a Name?" we discover that just as the definition of compassion is multifaceted, so too is the meaning of fatigue. Fatigue is most easily understood as extreme exhaustion after a particular activity. Each of us can remember how exhausted we felt when we moved from one house to another. After the movers left, we plopped on the coach and every muscle of our body screamed for attention. Although it might be difficult to acknowledge, the daily work of caregiving is often exhausting.

Sometimes the fatigue is physical, and our bodies ache because of the demands of the day. Social psychologist Christina Maslach explained the symptoms can be physical, emotional, and spiritual: "Symptoms of physical exhaustion can be somatic complaints, weight loss or weight gain, gastric intestinal distress, insomnia, and aches and pains just to name a few."[149]

Other times, we are emotionally exhausted because we witnessed a specific traumatic event or experienced vicarious trauma because of something a patient or client disclosed to us. Signs of emotional fatigue can be emotional outbursts, emotional instability, anger, suicidal ideation, cynicism, irritability, racing thoughts, sarcasm, poor concentration, violent fantasies, excessive fear, panic, and anxiety. When the symptoms of compassion fatigue start rearing their ugly heads, we may isolate ourselves and deprive ourselves of supportive relationships. Relationship problems, isolation, troubled relationships with coworkers, and fears of sharing one's experience with another are examples of experiencing relationship fatigue. Instead of turning toward a loved one or colleague, we isolate ourselves, possibly even self-medicating with drugs, alcohol, gambling, sex, and food.[150]

Of equal importance, our spiritual values may be challenged. We seem to be drifting out to sea, experiencing a loss of meaning and purpose, caught in a riptide where our spiritual values seem to get lost. Caregivers experience a loss of joy and happiness. They become like robots, showing up at work to do a job but without the passion they once had. We all know through our experiences with peers that some members are on the precipice of falling into compassion fatigue.

Another form of fatigue is called burnout. Maslach defined burnout as "a psychological syndrome of emotional exhaustion, depersonalization, and reduced personal accomplishment."[151] There is an uncanny similarity between Maslach's definition and the earlier definition by Freudenberger, who identified burnout as "a state of fatigue or frustration brought about by devotion to a cause, or way of life, or to a particular relationship that fails to produce an expected reward."[152] Gentry and Baranosky (1998) captured the essence of burnout as "The chronic condition of perceived demands outweighing perceived outcomes."[153]

Where to Begin?

If compassion fatigue and burnout are a danger to caregivers, and if the very art of caregiving presupposes we will experience pain and suffering, then how do we build the needed resiliency to protect ourselves? The easiest answer is one step at a time. The first is to become aware of—not afraid of—the symptoms. We cannot just expect the symptoms will go away on their own. The opposite is true. They will become worse and may lead to work interruption, absenteeism, and loss of productivity. How do we become comfortable in our own skin, learning to welcome, learning to become hospitable to those stirrings of the Soul, to the Soul pain that screams for attention? Recently, two of my clients were struggling with the cultural notion that they must do everything themselves. Both are overwhelmed, both have friends willing to help, and both have an ingrained stubbornness about seeking any help. Interestingly, as I felt the compassion of Leo, so too are each of these clients responding to the compassion I have for them.

How do we, as caregivers, respond to the loving invitations from family, friends, and colleagues knocking gently at our door? The first step is to listen to those stirrings, and if we don't hear them, can we trust a loving person to mirror them to us? This is one of the first steps Gentry suggested in his presentation of the three skills that are effective in resolving current symptoms of complex compassion fatigue and to prevent future effects.[154] The first is to admit to oneself that there is an issue requiring your attention. Soul has its way to breaking down the barriers that block us from listening to Soul Pain. You will recall my experience of breaking down when making spaghetti sauce for a company retreat. I had had enough. Like an addict lying in the gutter, realizing another "fix" would not help, or trying to get the last drop of booze from an empty whiskey bottle, I had reached the point of no return. I had to trust the interior movements of my soul. I had to take the risk of seeking help. I could no longer do this on my own.

The second step is to connect with a friend, family member, coach, counselor, or colleague for support. Simply ask them if they could listen to what is stirring and may be causing anguish in your Soul. Remind them that listening is not giving advice. If you are afraid of their reaction, pause for a moment, take a deep breath, and take the risk. This is the natural hesitancy, and sometimes fear, that accompanies vulnerability, which may be a new experience for you. You may gently tell them they don't need to solve or fix anything. You just want them to listen, which may be new for them. Certainly, it is reasonable for you to also reach out to a coach, pastor, or counselor. Being able to articulate your inner stirrings, as best you can, is already a step on the road to recovery.

I like Terri Lonowski's approach to listening, which is called Soulful Listening.[155] In her work, Lonoski addresses the cultural epidemic of loneliness. So many people are on social media, yet they feel isolated and disconnected from personal human interaction. Massive business closures due to the COVID-19 pandemic have only exacerbated this epidemic of isolation. We're too busy to call, so we text instead. We're too busy to write a note, so forget to say "thank you" or even send a quick email. Fortunately, Lonowski stresses that social isolation can be overcome through Soulful Listening. Simply put, these two words capture the art of listening and the goal of this book. She suggested five different practices of Soulful Listening for overcoming loneliness: developing self-care skills, becoming fully present, developing empathy and active listening skills, inspired action, and providing a feedback loop. I share Lonowski's understanding of self-care as a deep dive, hence the inclusion of the word Soul. Self-care is a daily practice and part of a daily routine which allows people to be fully present with each other and with themselves. Becoming present with oneself and with others requires us to be fully aware of the here and now. As discussed earlier, this requires a hospitality of the heart.

An attitude of empathy, coupled with active listening, makes the other person feel that you really care about them. When someone does not feel heard, they feel discounted and unappreciated. Inspired action is a practice to not only care for oneself but also to reach out to others. Rediscovering one's Soul and assisting another to rediscover their own has its own reward. Finally, Lonowski describes the "Feedback Loop."[156] This component of Soulful Listening requires us to act on the behalf of the other, and then communicate to them that we have acted for their benefit, which Lonowski says builds confidence and empowers the other. Lonowski's Soulful Listening allows the caregiver to take the risk of what can be called rooted flight, where one is grounded and at the same time able to fly. Taking the risk also necessitates addressing one's Soul Pain.

Those in pain need to break the silence and take the risk to seek help, as well as be open to those who care about you and offer to help. We always answer automatically we hear the greeting "Hello, how are you doing?" We say "Fine," even when we feel awful. "Fine" allows us to acknowledge the other person and be on our way. I love the Italian greeting, "Come Sta" meaning "How are you?" and the possible responses, "Va bene," meaning "Very well," or "Non che Male," which can mean "There is no evil" or "I'm feeling sort of ok" or "Things could be worse." The greeting invites the greeter to ask more questions, and then the floodgates are opened.

As you reach out to someone, you are already entering into the realm of storytelling. What's the earliest memory you have of being told as story? Was it at a grandparent's house, or around a campfire at a Scout camp, or was it listening to a client in need? We all have stories to tell, so it's not that we have to rack our brain for one. Most of them are on the tip of our tongues. When was the last time you felt that someone was really interested in what you had to say? Stories allow us to reflect, and to envision new possibilities.

Storytelling becomes a powerful means of looking at oneself from a safe and alternative perspective. The stories throughout this work have been gleaned from personal interviews and experiences. These stories encompassed experiences of grief, PTSD, and compassion fatigue. There were stories of complex family relationships, sexual abuse, auto accidents, exceptional caregiving, a physician's compassion, significant life transitions, a chaplain's interventions, the dance of caregiving with two twin brothers, a professor as mentor, and a nurse's compassion with a dying person.

At the end of each chapter in this book, there are reflection questions which are often about the stories in the chapter. I hope that one or two of these questions struck home and allowed you to pause and reflect. I hope you are inspired to journal and create a story about yourself. There are no predetermined rules about how to tell a story. I'm sure you are already a pro (especially after a beer or two). Nothing but your willingness to tell your story is required. No preamble. Just start writing or start talking. Someone wants to hear your story, and as you relate it, either verbally or in writing, you will discover that the story becomes a mirror which reflects the real you.

The third skill that helps lessen and alleviate the symptoms of compassion fatigue is creating a practice of relaxation. We have the luxury of time, and it is possible to find designated spaces in one's day, week, or month for reflection and relaxation. Do you have time to take a quiet walk each day, perhaps before or after work? Have you wanted to take a cooking class or sign up for a writing group or a hiking club? What about reading that European travel guide or taking the fishing trip you always put off? Are you willing to go to that workshop on centering prayer and learn more about your spirituality? Do you have or want to develop a spiritual practice? Can you pause and reflect on who and what is meaningful to you?

How many times have you had time for relaxation, enrichment, or reflection, only to rationalize them away, convincing yourself you are simply too busy? If you avoid spending time on what brings you joy and inspiration, it's time to start listening to the stirrings of your Soul. This process can begin simply, such as planning a new weekly activity, but the long-term effects of taking time for yourself are profound.

Recovery from the symptoms of compassion fatigue is possible, and when you do recover, you will learn how to avoid falling into compassion fatigue and burnout in the future. These three practices help us develop a resilience that allows us to be faithful to the original call to be a caregiver, where we find meaning and spiritual support. We can continue to have a passion for our work because our caregiving defines who we are. In allowing ourselves to be vulnerable, we rediscover the value of those who support and sustain us, and in doing so, we strengthen these relationships. Each step forward helps us steadily gain self-confidence and resilience in times of stress.

Resting Places Along the Way

In summary, the caregiver's guide is not something external to us but is internal. It is not a "How-To" book, but rather, a journey in discovering and reclaiming our Soul. We explored the dance of caregiving, the meaning of listening to the Soul, the mythos of our vocation, the art of hospitality, the reality of our limitations, the sacredness of our work, the exhausting nature of compassion, and the need to develop compassion resilience.

The caregiver reading this book becomes a pilgrim, and each chapter is like a new oasis to explore, as well as a place to ponder and rest in the landscape of the Soul. Rest wherever you need time to ponder and reflect. There is no rush. If need be, continue and join the next pilgrimage. Feel free to hop on or off, as you need to, there is always another pilgrimage passing through your current rest stop.

Trust your insights. You know because you know. Take the risk that will enliven you. Listen to where your Soul wishes to take you, then go there. And most importantly, enjoy the journey.

A Moment of Reflection

At your own pace, give yourself a moment to reflect on each question below.

1. Has the idea that compassion fatigue is a normal outcome for caregivers surprised you?

2. Do you currently have any symptoms of compassion fatigue, and if so, what steps can you take to help yourself?

3. Because you are a caregiver, you will necessarily be drawn into the mystery of pain and suffering. How will you cultivate and maintain compassion resilience in your caregiving work?

_____

_____

_____

_____

_____

_____

_____

_____

_____

_____

_____

_____

Just when the
caterpillar
thought the
world
was over,
it became
a butterfly.

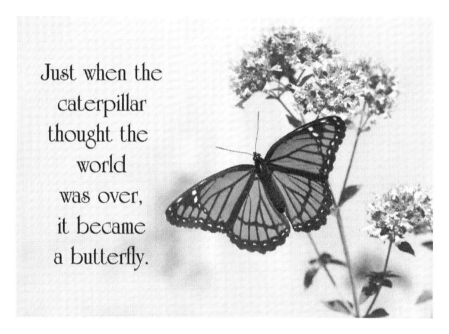

Postscript

Endings and Beginnings

There is a finality in saying "The End." But that is where we are. This is the end of the *Soul of Caregiving*. As you read, you learned about *THE DANCE* of caregiving, which balances caring for others with care of the self. You risked going deeper through reflection in order to rediscover *SOUL*, the force that animates and grounds you. You found the balance between *CREATIVITY* and *REASON*. Your gift of caregiving was strengthened when you rediscovered its *ARCHETYPAL* nature. The welcoming arms of *HOSPITALITY* surrounded you and taught you that your story needs to be told and heard. You were relieved to learn you don't have to be perfect because we are all *WOUNDED HEALERS*. You were surprised to learn *REFLECTION* is a normal human activity. You remembered your caregiving work has a sacred, *SPIRITUAL* dimension. Your insights will mature through your *PRACTICE* of caregiving. And learning you can *RECOVER* from compassion fatigue was the greatest insight of all.

Did I say this was the end? Well, it is, but every ending is a new beginning. You have crossed a threshold into the land of possibility. Insights borne from your Soul will continue to nourish and support you as you develop the skills of self-care and compassion resilience. And if the focus of your journey was your own recovery, I hope you reach out to other caregivers seeking similar support. Your ability to share your journey may give other caregivers the courage to take the first step to recovery.

Caring for Caregivers

In her review of the first edition of *The Soul of Caregiving*, Dr. Carol S. Pearson mentioned that caregivers are often misunderstood and underpaid; they are not appropriately honored or given the respect that they truly deserve. In her review for this revised edition, Dr. Pearson observed that "Even today, our survival is dependent upon this, yet caregivers are often taken for granted. Much of caregiving is done in our homes and communities without pay, and many in caring fields are underpaid and/or over worked. But now, our current pandemic has challenged all of us to show our care for one another by being vaccinated and wearing masks, and our heroes are those who are the essential workers who care for the sick and for the survival needs of all of us."

We need to support caregivers, perhaps now more than ever before. This support can take many forms, but I think the most important thing is to simply listen and be there for them. They don't want advice, just to be heard. Being present and listening to their story is the greatest gift you can give. Explore options in your community to support caregivers as best you can and encourage others to do the same. You have so much to give.

Thank you for caring for yourself by taking the time to rediscover the many gifts you bring and the gift you are. If you are ready to explore the possibility of coaching, visit my website (SoulofCaregiving.com). Please consider also writing a review about your experience and my book on Amazon.

Dr. Edward M. Smink

About the Author

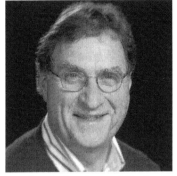

Dr. Edward M. Smink, Ph.D. has over forty years of experience in healthcare as nurse, crisis and pastoral counselor, executive leader, facilitator of mission, ethics, value and leadership formation and community health. He served on local, regional and international committees of value formation in the United States, Australia, Korea, England, Spain and Italy. His career of coaching has the foundation of his many years in different leadership positions where his skills of active listening, the promotion of ethical and professional guidelines, crisis intervention, facilitation of personal and professional goals, growth strategies, and sensitivity for and the promotion of cultural and spiritual diversity has taught him much wisdom.

Edward likes to claim that along with his academic credentials, he has learned most from his experience with colleagues who care for others and from those who needed his services. Edward's focus on coaching includes an emphasis on the development of strengths and the integration of values in personal and professional practice. He is passionate about the universal values and archetypes that unite humankind and with his background in mythological studies, enjoys discovering the unique personal stories of each client that contribute to successful outcomes. More information about Dr. Edward M. Smink can be found on his website:

www.SoulofCaregiving.com

References

[1] Carteret, Marcia. "Cultural Differences in Family Dynamics." *Dimensions of Culture: Cross-Cultural Communications for Healthcare Professionals*, Smashwords, 2012.

[2] Kearney, Michael. *Mortally Wounded: Stories of Soul Pain, Death and Healing*. Touchstone, Simon and Schuster, 1996.

[3] ---. *Mortally Wounded: Stories of Soul Pain, Death, and Healing*. Touchstone, Simon and Schuster, 1996.

[4] Hillman, James. *The Dream and the Underworld*. Harper and Row, 1979. (p. x.)

[5] Moore, Thomas. *Care of the Soul*. Harper, 1992.

[6] ---. *The Dream and the Underworld*. Harper and Row, 1979.

[7] Hillman, James. *The Thought of the Heart and the Soul of the World*. Spring, 1992.

[8] Kearney, Michael. *Mortally Wounded: Stories of Soul Pain, Death and Healing*. Touchstone, Simon and Schuster, 1996.

[9] Lencioni, Patrick. *Five Dysfunctions of a Team*. Jossey-Bass. 2002.

[10] Simon and Garfunkel. "The 59th Street Bridge Song." *Parsley, Sage, Rosemary and Thyme*. 1966.

[11] Romanyshyn, Robert. *The Ways of the Heart: Essays Toward an Imaginal Psychology*. Trivium, 2002.

[12] Avens, Robert. *Imagination is Reality: Western Nirvana in Jung, Hillman, Barfield and Cassirer*. Spring Publications, 2003.

[13] Ulanov, Anne and Barry. *The Healing Imagination: The Meeting of Psyche and Soul*. Daimon Verlag, 2000.

[14] Jung, Carl Gustav. "A Psychological Approach to the Trinity." *The Collected Works of C. G. Jung*. Vol. 11. Translated by R.F.C. Hull. Princeton University Press, 1977.

[15] Ibid.

[16] Pearson, Carol. *Awakening the Heroes Within: Twelve Archetypes to Help Us Find Ourselves and Transform Our World*. HarperOne, 2015

[17] Woodman, Marion. *Addiction to Perfection*. Inner City Books, 1982

[18] Wegscheider-Cruse, Sharon. "6 Common Roles in an Addicted Household [Blog]." *American Addiction Centers*. https://rehabs.com/blog/6-common-family-roles-in-an-addicted-household/ Nov. 2019

[19] Ibid.

[20] National Center for PTSD. https://www.ptsd.va.gov/understand/what/ptsd_basics.asp. July, 2021.

[21] Ibid.

[22] Atlee, Cindy et al. The Storybranding Group. To learn more visit https://www.storybranding.com/about/ July 2021.

[23] Jung, Carl Gustav. "On the Relation of Analytical Psychology to Poetry." *The Collected Works of C. G. Jung*, Vol. 15. Translated by R.F.C. Hull. Princeton University Press, 1981.

[24] Kosslyn, Stephen M. and Miller, G. Wayne. "Left Brain, Right Brain: Two Sides, Always Working Together." *Psychology Today*. May 7, 2014.

[25] Hillman, James. *The Soul's Code.* Warner Books, 1996.

[26] Oglesby, Pamela. "Right Brain vs Left Brain Functions." www.owlcation.com/socialscience, 2017.

[27] Musgrove, Becky. "Right Vs. Left Brain: Which Rules You?" www.lifescript.com.

[28] McQuerrey, Lisa. "What are Good People Skills." Chron.com.

[29] International Coaching Federation. "Core Competencies." https://coachfederation.org/credential/compentencies.

[30] Press Ganey. Patient Experience Solutions. https://www.pressganey.com/solutions/patient-experience.

[31] Jaucourt, Louis chevalier de. "Hospitalité." *The Encyclopedia of Diderot & Alembert Collaborative Translation Project*. Translated by Sophie Bourgault. University of Michigan Library, 2013.

[32] Sunil, Amitabh Kant. *Branding India: An Incredible Story*. HarperCollins Publishers India, 2009.

[33] Mandelbaum, Allen. *The Metamorphosis of Ovid*. Book VIII, 273-277. Harcourt, Brace, & Co., 1993.

[34] McKenzie, John L. Dictionary of the Bible. "Hospitality." Geoffrey Chapman, 1976.

[35] Luke 7:36-50. *The New Oxford Annotated Bible 3rd Edition*. Oxford University Press, 2001.

[36] Acts 14:11-12. *The New Oxford Annotated Bible 3rd Edition*. Oxford University Press, 2001.

[37] Hebrews 13:2. *The New Oxford Annotated Bible 3rd Edition*. Oxford University Press, 2001.

[38] Augsburger, William. *Pastoral Counseling Across Cultures*, Westminster, 1986.

[39] Madelina, Sister. CSJ. Hospitality Poster. Sisters of St. Joseph of Orange, CA

[40] US Department of State. "Active Listening." https://www.state.gov/m/a/os/65759.html.

[41] Madelina, Sister. CSJ. Hospitality Poster. Sisters of St. Joseph of Orange, CA

[42] Psalm 139. *The New Oxford Annotated Bible 3rd Edition*. Oxford University Press, 2001.

[43] Campbell, Joseph. *Thou Art That*. Edited by Eugene Kennedy. New World Library, 2001.

[44] McMahon, Norbert. *The Story of the Hospitallers of St. John of God*. M.H. Gill & Son, 1958.

[45] McKenzie, John L. *The Dictionary of the Bible*. "Grace." Geoffrey Chapman, 1976.

[46] Arrien, Angeles. "The Healing Encounter*." Care for the Journey: Messages and Music for Sustaining the Heart of Healthcare*. Companion Arts, 2005.

[47] Puchalski, Christina. The Healing Encounter." *Care for the Journey: Messages and Music for Sustaining the Heart of Healthcare*. Companion Arts, 2005.

[48] Smink, E.M. "Theology of Pastoral Care." *Certification Papers*. National Association of Catholic Chaplains, 1991.

[49] Augsburger, William. Pastoral Counseling Across Cultures, Westminster, 1986.

[50] Guggenbühl-Craig, Adolph. *Power in the Healing Professions*. Spring, 1971.

[51] Jung, Carl Gustav. *Memories, Dreams, Reflections*. Edited by Aniela Jaffe. Vintage Books, 1989.

[52] Hampel, Patricia. *I Could Tell You Stories: Sojourns in the Land of Memory*. W. W. Norton, 1999.

[53] Slattery, Dennis P. *The Wounded Body, Remembering the Markings of Flesh*. SUNY Press, 2000.

[54] McKean, Erin, editor. *The Oxford American Dictionary and Thesaurus*. "Selfish." Oxford University Press, 2003.

[55] Jung, Carl Gustav. "The Psychology of the Transference." *The Collected Works of C. G. Jung*, Vol. 16, Translated by R. F. C. Hull. Princeton University Press, 1985.

[56] Campbell, Joseph. *The Hero with a Thousand Faces*. Bollingen Series XVII. Pantheon, 1949.

[57] Hillman, James. *Re-Visioning Psychology*. Harper Colophon, 1975.

[58] Morrison, Toni. "Memory, Creation, and Writing." *Anatomy of Memory*, edited by James McConkey. Oxford University Press, 1996.

[59] Downing, Christine. "Only the Wounded Healer Heals: The Testimony of Greek Mythology." *Soundings 73.4*, 1990.

[60] ---. *The Hero with a Thousand Faces*.

[61] Brazier, Yvetter. "Why was Medieval Islamic Medicine So Important?" *Medical News Today*. November 9, 2018.

[62] Groesbeck, C. J. "The Archetypal Image of the Wounded Healer." *Journal of Analytical Psychology*, vol. 20, issue 2, 1975, pp. 122-145.

[63] Matthews, Thomas F. *The Clash of the Gods: A Reinterpretation of Early Christian Art.* Princeton University Press, 1993.

[64] Kerényi, Carl. Asklepios: *Archetypal Image of the Physician' Existence,* edited by Ralph Manheim. Bollingen Series LXV. Vol. 3. Princeton University Press, 1981.

[65] Nouwen, Henri, J. M. *The Wounded Healer*. Doubleday, 1993.

[66] Ba-Hunas, Ilyas. "Al-Faregui and beyond: Future Trends in Islamization of Knowledge." *The American Journal of Islamic Science*, Vol.5, 1988.

[67] ---. "Why was Medieval Islamic Medicine So Important?"

[68] "The Significance of Ibn Sina's Canon of Medicine in the Arab and Western worlds." *Science and Its Times: Understanding the Social Significance of Scientific Discovery.* https://www.encyclopedia.com/science/encyclopedias-almanacs-transcripts-and-maps/significance-ibn-sinas-canon-medicine-arab-and-western-worlds.

[69] ---. "Why was Medieval Islamic Medicine So Important?"

[70] von Eschenbach, Wolfram. *Parzival*. Penguin Books, 1980.

[71] Chevalier, Jean and Alain Gheerbrant. *The Penguin Book of Symbols.* Translated by John Buchanan-Brown. Pantheon, 1996.

[72] Hillman, James. *The Thought of the Heart and the Soul of the World.* Spring, 1992.

[73] ---. *The Thought of the Heart and the Soul of the World.*

[74] ---. *The Hero with a Thousand Faces*.

[75] Campbell, Joseph. *The Masks of God: Creative Mythology*. Penguin, 1968.

[76] De Castro, Francisco. "The First Biography of St. John of God." Translated by Benedict O'Grady. Secretariat for the English Language Provinces of the Order, 1986.

[77] Doniger O'Flaherty, Wendy. "Inside and Outside the Mouth of God: The Boundary between Myth and Reality." *Daedalus*, vol. 109, no. 2, 1980.

[78] ---. *Memories, Dreams, Reflections*.

[79] Sperry, Len. "Holistic Treatment of the Wounded Healer: Medical, Psychological, and Pastoral Aspects." *Individual Psychology,* vol. 43, no. 4, 1987, pp. 538-541.

[80] Daneault, Serge. 'The Wounded Healer: Can This Idea Be of Use to Family Physicians?" *Canadian Family Physician*, vol. 54, no. 9, 2008, pp. 1218-1219.

[81] Ibid.

[82] ---. "Only the Wounded Healer Heals: The Testimony of Greek Mythology." *Soundings 73.4*, 1990.

[83] Bridges, William. *Transitions: Making Sense of Life's Changes*. Da Capo Press, 2004.

[84] Ibid.

[85] *Children of a Lesser God*. Paramount Pictures, 1986.

[86] Merton, Thomas. *The Hidden Ground of Love: Letters*. Edited by. William Shannon. Farrar, Straus, Giroux, 1985. Letter 438 and Letter 621.

[87] ---. *The Healing Imagination: The Meeting of Psyche and Soul*.

[88] Luke 13, 6-9: "A man had a fig tree planted in his vineyard, and he came looking for some fruit on it and found none. So, he said to the gardener, 'See here! For three years I have come looking for fruit on this fig tree, still I fine none. Cut it down! Why should it be wasting the soil?' He replied, 'Sir, let it alone for one more year until I dig around it and put manure on it. If it bears fruit next year, well and good; but if not, you can cut it down.'" from *The New Oxford Annotated Bible*, Oxford University Press, 2001.

[89] Harding, Mary Esther. *Psychic Energy: Its Source and Transformation*. Princeton University Press, 1973.

[90] Bosnak, Robert. *Embodiment: Creative Imagination in Medicine, Art, and Travel*. Routledge, 2008.

[91] Poole Heller, Diane. *Crash Course*. North Atlantic Books, 2001.

[92] Ibid.

93 Campbell, Joseph. *The Flight of the Wild Gander*. New World Library, 2004.

94 Nuland, Sherwin B. *How We Die*. Alfred A. Knopf, 1944.

95 Koenig Harold G. "Religion, Spirituality, and Medicine: Application to Clinical Practice." *JAMA*. vol. 284, no. 13, 2000, p. 1708.

96 Koenig, Harold G. et al. *Handbook of Religion and Health*, 2nd ed., Oxford University Press, 2012.

97 Koenig, Harold G. "The relationship between religious activities and blood pressure in older adults." International Journal Psychiatry in Medicine, vol. 28, no. 2, 1998, 189-213.

98 Smith, Houston. *The Illustrated World's Religions: A Guide to Our Wisdom Traditions*. Harper, 1994.

99 Egendorf, A. "Hearing people through their pain." *Journal of Traumatic Stress*, vol. 8, no.1, 1995, 5-28.

100 May, Rollo. *Care of Mind/Care of Spirit*. Harper and Row, 1982.

101 ---. *Thou Art That*.

102 Ibid.

103 Corbett, Lionel. *The Religious Function of the Psyche*. Routledge, 1996.

104 Bettelheim, Bruno. *Freud and Man's Soul*. Vintage, 1986.

105 ---. "The Psychology of the Transference," pp. 230-231.

106 Grant, Robert. *The Way of the Wound: A Spirituality of Trauma and Transformation*. Robert Grant, 1997.

107 Pearson, C., et al. *The Storybranding Group*. https://www.storybranding.com/

108 Greenleaf, Robert K. *Servant Leadership*. Paulist Press, 1977.

109 ---. *The Storybranding Group*.

110 The Balm of Gilead is interpreted as a spiritual medicine that heals Israel (and sinners in general). In *The Old Testament*, the balm of Gilead is taken most directly from Jeremiah 8: 22.

111 Smith, Patricia. *To Weep for the Stranger: Compassion Fatigue in Caregiving*. Create Space, 2009.

112 Berry, Thomas. *The Dream of the Earth*. Sierra, 1988.

113 Campbell, Joseph. *Transformations of Myth through Time*. Vol. 1, Tape 5. High Bridge Productions, 1990.

114 Sing, K.V. *Hindu Rites and Rituals: Origins and Meanings*. Penguin Books, 2015.

[115] Campbell, Joseph. *The Inner Reaches of Outer Space: Metaphor as Myth and Religion*. New World Library, 2002.

[116] Paden, William, E. *Interpreting the Sacred: Ways of Viewing Religion*. Beacon, 1992.

[117] ---. *Memories, Dreams, Reflections*.

[118] ---. *The Way of the Wound: A Spirituality of Trauma and Transformation*.

[119] Jung, Carl Gustav. *Mysterium Coniunctionis*. Translated by R. F. C. Hull. *The Collected Works of C. G. Jung*, vol. 20. Princeton University Press, 1977, p. 330.

[120] .---. *Re-Visioning Psychology*.

[121] Mogenson, Greg. *A Most Accursed Religion: When Trauma becomes a God*. Spring, 2005.

[122] Ibid.

[123] Association of American Medical Colleges. "Report III, Contemporary Issues in Medicine: Communication in Medicine." Medical School Objectives Project, October 1999. https://www.aamc.org/media/24236/download.

[124] Ibid.

[125] Moore, Thomas. "The Soul of Medicine," *Spirituality and Health*, vol 9, no. 3, 2006, 10-11.

[126] Haque, Amber and Hooman Keshavarzi. "Integrating indigenous healing methods in therapy: Muslim beliefs and practices." *International Journal of Culture and Mental Health*, vol. 7, no. 3, 2014, 297-314.

[127] Clift, Jean Dalby, and Wallace B. Clift. *The Archetype of Pilgrimage: Outer Action with Inner Meaning*. Paulist, 1996.

[128] Niebuhr, Richard R. "Pilgrims and Pioneers." *Parabola*, vol. 9, no. 3, 1984, 6-13.

[129] Johnson, Robert A. *Inner Work*. Harper & Row, 1986.

[130] ---. *The Hero with a Thousand Faces*.

[131] Maslach, Christina. *Burnout: The Cost of Caring*. Jossey-Bass, 1982.

[132] ---. *To Weep for the Stranger: Compassion Fatigue in Caregiving*.

[133] ---. *Parzival*.

[134] Ibid.

[135] Figley, Charles. *Compassion Fatigue*. Routledge, 1995.

[136] Gawande, Atul. *The Checklist Manifesto: How to Get Things Right*. Metropolitan, 2009.

[137] Nouwen, Henri J. M., et al. *Compassion A Reflection on the Christian Life.* Darton, Longman, Todd, 2008.

[138] Gentry, Eric. Certification Training for Compassion Fatigue Professionals (CCFP). https://catalog.pesi.com/sales/bh_c_045740_ccfp_organic-16508. January 2018.

[139] Küng, Hans. *Global Responsibility: In Search of a New World Ethic.* Wipf and Stock, 2004.

[140] Bakker, Freek L. "Comparing the Golden Rule in Hindu and Christian Religious Texts." *Studies in Religion/Sciences Religieuses,* vol. 42, no. 1, 2012, 38-58.

[141] Lampert, Khen. *Traditions of Compassion: From Religious Duty to Social Activism.* Macmillan, 2006.

[142] Elias, Abu Amina. "The Golden Rule in Islam." *Islamic Information Portal.* http://islam.ru/en/content/story/golden-rule-islam. 26 Feb. 2013.

[143] Schaaf. Gregory. "From the Great Law of Peace to the Constitution of the United States: A Revision of America's Democratic Roots." *American Indian Law Review,* vol. 14, no. 2, 1988/1989, University Press of Oklahoma College of Law.

[144] Lander, Lorne. *The Lost Art of Compassion.* HarperCollins, 2004.

[145] Ibid.

[146] ---. *The Wounded Healer.*

[147] ---. *Memories, Dreams, Reflections.*

[148] Maslach, Christina & Michael Leiter. *The Truth About Burnout: How Organizations Cause Personal Stress and What to do about it.* Jossey-Bass, 1997.

[149] ---. *Burnout: The Cost of Caring.*

[150] ---. "Become a Certified Compassion Fatigue Professional."

[151] ---. Certification Training for Compassion Fatigue Professionals (CCFP).

[152] ---. *Burnout: The Cost of Caring.*

[153] Freudenberger, Herbert J., and Geraldine Richelson. *Burnout: The High Cost of High Achievement.* Anchor Press, 1980.

[154] Gentry, J., & Baranowsky, A. *Treatment manual for the Accelerated Recovery Program: Set II.* Psych Ink, 1998.

[155] Ibid.

[156] Georgiadis, Fortis. "Terri Lonowski: 5 Things We Can Each Do Held Solve The Loneliness Epidemic." https://medium.com/authority-magazine/terri-lonowski-5-things-we-can-each-do-help-solve-the-loneliness-epidemic-7671b34375ba. October 27, 2020.

Made in the USA
Las Vegas, NV
27 October 2021